The Reactive Hypoglycemia Sourcebook

Second Edition

Stephanie Kenrose

ISBN 978-1460916964

Cover art by Thomas Perkins

Contents

Chapter 1: Introduction

"Generalized anxiety disorder." That's the diagnosis I received from my general practitioner when I was 28 years old after several years of vague symptoms. That added another ailment to my growing list. My physicians and psychologists always had an answer for my mystifying health problems. My mania, they said, was due to bipolar disorder. My lethargy was due to depression, my palpitations were due to panic attacks (even when my heartbeat was beating at a normal 70 beats per minute), my fainting was because of low blood pressure, my failure to lose weight was caused by to incorrect eating habits and not enough exercise (as a vegetarian exercising 40 minutes a day I didn't think I quite fit *that* profile), my hot and cold spells—where my limbs would shiver at times then at other times I'd heat up like a furnace—were a result of early menopause. Despite all the modern miracles of drugs and years of psychotherapy, I never got better, and in fact, got worse.

I was a physical and emotional wreck. Sometimes, I would stay in bed for days.

My three pregnancies all ended in a 60-pound weight gain. I craved carbs like a crack addict. Nothing but French fries and chocolate cake could stop me feeling deathly sick; my body refused to eat salad, and if I forced myself to eat anything healthy, I threw it up. Diagnosed with hyperemesis, I spend most of my pregnancies throwing up chunks and laying in bed, too nauseas to move an inch. It was like I was on a permanent Wurlitzer flinging me into the land of nausea and malaise.

After a bout of the flu in 2005, I went to my doctor complaining of persistent malaise; I couldn't walk ten feet without being exhausted. My blood pressure had dropped to 70/60. An armful of glucose raised my blood pressure to normal levels again. The next day, I felt ready to run a marathon. It wasn't long before I got sick again. With bi-monthly bouts of "gastroenteritis" or lactose intolerance. I felt constantly stressed, despite a magically happy home life and a low-stress job as a part time mathematics professor. There was nothing to cause me stress. Nothing, that is, except my "bipolar" disorder, my "generalized anxiety disorder" and my "early menopause."

As I struggled with my weight, all of my physicians recommended that I lose a few pounds, but none of them recommended a trip to the dietician. If I had gone to see a dietician, and told her my diet, that may have put me on the road to recovery. Although I was a vegetarian and considered myself a healthy eater, I know now that my diet consisted of many of the "wrong" kinds of foods: white rice, potatoes, chocolate cake, chocolate bars, candy (I was addicted to an English candy), high-sugar fruits like bananas and orange juice, and six cups of coffee a day.

My ex-husband tried to get me to quit caffeine, and we would have a "see who can cite the most research" competition. He would produce the latest news on why caffeine had been linked to numerous health problems. I would drag up articles suggesting caffeine caused *no* health problems. If only had I know at the time that caffeine is to reactive hypoglycemics what chocolate cake is to diabetics.

Reactive hypoglycemia is often misdiagnosed as "stress," bipolar disorder, generalized anxiety disorder, and personality disorder.

My son, Leo, also began to show symptoms of the same kind, only his "fainting" resulted in Grand Mal seizures. I asked my physician about fainting and seizures. "We have the same symptoms," I said. "But when Leo passes out, he has a seizure, and I don't." "Seizures aren't always visible," my physician said. "Someone could be looking you in the eye and be having a seizure and you wouldn't even know it." I recalled my brother-in-law, Gary. He had Tourette's, and when he had a seizure, he would contort his mouth like a dog chewing a spoonful of peanut butter. That was usually the only sign that something was wrong.

My poor ex-husband was often the recipient of mood swings, not only from me, but from Leo as well. Sometimes I would be irritable to the point of not being able to speak. Sometimes Leo would slam doors so hard he would break the hinges. Sometimes I would be "depressed" to the point of not being able to speak, and sometimes Leo would hurl himself onto his bed in the middle of the afternoon and sleep for hours. "You're always sick," my husband said. My best friend said it too. "Six bouts of food poisoning in one year *not* normal," she said. No, it wasn't normal. But perhaps, I convinced myself, I was just unlucky. Perhaps I had been the one to touch the E-Coli contaminated surface just before I ate, or perhaps I was the unfortunate one that got the moldy serving of peas, or maybe my body was simply just more susceptible to stomach ailments.

I began to suspect some kind of immune disorder. HIV? Multiple Sclerosis? Thyroid disease? Chediak-Higashi syndrome? Chronic granulomatous disease? I must have spent months researching every odd disease known to man, becoming an expert on strange and unusual disease. Some of them sounded close, but none sounded exactly right. Then one morning I found a post on a health discussion board.

"Please help. For months I've been suffering from feeling so dizzy or lightheaded I felt like I would pass out, but I don't. This is in combination with feeling extremely nauseas accompanied by very bad diarrhea. It comes out of the blue. I could just be sitting watching a movie and it will happen. It's so disjointed a feeling; it's hard to put into words what I feel like. Sometimes it feels like the flu, or gastric flu, or food poisoning, or…something else that produces hot and cold chills."

A shiver ran down my spine. I thought that I could have written that post. I read on, through a lengthy discussion where many people reported the same kinds of symptoms. Another board poster replied "have you looked into reactive hypoglycemia?" And that is where my journey really began.

I began to research reactive hypoglycemia intensively. Although I'm not a physician (in fact, I teach college mathematics and my knowledge of the practice of medicine is limited to an undergrad degree in pre-med), I learned how to conduct diligent research while in grad school. After I had sifted through many popular articles on the web (most of which had blatantly incorrect information), I learned that reactive hypoglycemia doesn't usually lead to more serious consequences (reactive hypoglycemia rarely has complications like my son's seizures, and mortality is never seen).[1] I also learned that a failure to understand and treat this disease can lead to serious consequences, like delayed reactions when driving a car or operating heavy machinery. Seeing as I commuted an hour and a half once a week to a state university at the time, I thought that I should perhaps take this advice seriously, and began packing snacks and drinks with me on the trip. At times when my symptoms were at their worst, I had difficulty driving: I felt anxious, jittery, and once I drove into a shopping cart (I am very thankful it was a cart and not a person). And yet, my doctor insisted there was nothing physically wrong with me, and my experiences were yet again chalked down to "stress."

In an article in Diabetes Metabolism, Researcher Jean-Frédéric Brun[2] stated that I am not alone; many physicians send patients complaining of reactive hypoglycemic symptoms to see a psychiatrist, even in recent years. The decades of doctors believing that reactive hypoglycemia as a "non-existent" disorder persists even today, and like OJ's reputation, may never quite recover.

A couple of months after my diagnosis of "stress," Leo's pediatrician diagnosed him with reactive hypoglycemia. I used an ambulatory blood glucose monitor to assist with my diagnosis (see chapter 4 for more on this test) for the same condition. Several months later, the seizures, the mood swings, the symptoms of "bipolar disorder" and "generalized anxiety disorder" and "stress" have all but disappeared. I can't remember the last time I had a heart palpitation, or had to run to the bathroom with a bout of diarrhea. Leo and I stopped eating simple carbs and sweets. Instead, we both went on a high-fiber, balanced vegan diet. Of course, it's not quite *that* simple, which is why I wrote this book.

* * *

The good news is that reactive hypoglycemia is now a known disease with definite symptoms and treatable causes. The trick to treating it is to first understand this elusive disorder, which has been called one of the "the great pretenders" of medicine because it mimics so many other diseases.

The Reactive Hypoglycemia Sourcebook is packed full of tips on how to diagnose & live with the condition. You'll find explanations of diagnostic tests, dietary tips, and dozens of references for further reading. And of course, you can always visit my blog at www.reactivehypoglycemia.info for links, recipes, a book store, and more. If you think you, or someone you know, has reactive hypoglycemia, this book was written for you.

Chapter 2: History

Part of the reason that doctors are sometimes inclined to ignore reactive hypoglycemia as a legitimate disorder is probably because of its rather checkered history in the medical establishment.

Reactive Hypoglycemia was first named as a disorder in 1924 by Dr. Seale Harris.[3] Until Harris's discovery, people with symptoms of hypoglycemia had often been diagnosed with coronary thrombosis, brain tumors, seizure disorders, alcoholism, and a host of other diseases and disorders. The disorder was controversial for decades afterward, mostly due to haphazard definitions and inappropriate tests.[4] A diagnosis of reactive hypoglycemia was an "in" diagnosis in the 1960s and 1970s, and alternative medicine practitioners blamed reactive hypoglycemia for almost every ailment possible, "curing" patients by prescribing a diet free of caffeine, alcohol, sugars, and simple carbohydrates.[5] The regular medical establishment was up in arms over the exploding number of cases of reactive hypoglycemia, and the term "pseudo hypoglycemia" to indicate that reactive hypoglycemia wasn't a "real" disease, or "reactive non hypoglycemia" to indicate that sometimes people thought they had reactive hypoglycemia when in fact they did not. There's no doubt that many people legitimately suffered from reactive hypoglycemia, but in the 60s and 70s, reliable tests didn't exist to weed out the people who had the disorder from those who didn't.

The over diagnosis of hypoglycemia spread like the swine flu, and soon became a worldwide phenomenon accompanied by an explosion of popular literature.[6] To add to the confusion, no one seemed to be able to settle on a term. Reactive hypoglycemia has been called a myriad of names including postrprandial reactive hypoglycemia, functional hyperinsulinism, functional hypoglycemia, and relative hypoglycemia.[7]

The failure of the clinical breakfast test to induce hypoglycemia[1] (see Chapter 4: Tests) led to one researcher concluding (in 1981) that reactive hypoglycemia didn't exist as a disease because of lack of evidence to support the disease's existence. The researcher's article, which appeared in issue 30 of *Diabetes*, said that hypoglycemia did not appear to be part of the syndrome (because they hadn't been able to reproduce low blood sugar in the lab). Thus, the term "idiopathic postprandial syndrome"[8] was born, and people with reactive hypoglycemia were assumed to have a reaction to food of unknown origin. Or to put it more simply, reactive hypoglycemia is not connected to blood sugar levels (and is most probably "all in the head"). The real problem may have been that a mixed meal breakfast test is too balanced and won't cause a reactive

---

[1] The Breakfast Test is no longer considered a valid method to measure for reactive hypoglycemia, because it fails to deliver the high-carb load that typically causes a hypoglycemic reaction.

hypoglycemic to experience the type of blood sugar drop people experience after they have after a high carbohydrate meal.[9]

Adding further to reactive hypoglycemia's reputation as a less than legitimate disease was its ability to mimic a host of other disorders, including seizure disorders, anxiety, depression, alcoholism, and behavior disorders. Sometimes, people with reactive hypoglycemia will even show an abnormal personality profile in a psychiatric exam.[10]

Diabetologists (medical doctors who specialize in diabetes) now know that reactive hypoglycemia can cause a wide variety of behavioral disturbances—there's even the suggestion that low blood sugar can cause schizophrenia.[11] It's also been associated with criminality, particularly

> Dan White, the man who assassinated Harvey Milk, was reactive hypoglycemic (at least, according to his defense lawyers). He was acquitted because his defense said his diet of sugary foods and drinks caused behavioral changes (the now famous "Twinkie Defense").

violent crime. The late morning, when prison inmates' blood sugar begins to drop, is a time typically associated with inmate violence.[12] Of course, just like not everyone with schizophrenia will have a delusion of being chased with men in red ties, not everyone with reactive hypoglycemia will experience violence, or even behavioral changes. The disorder has been linked to dozens of symptoms ranging from seizures to stomach upsets.

* * *

Up until a couple of decades ago, little was known about the physiology of reactive hypoglycemia; if you were suffering from the symptoms back then you would have been lucky to find a doctor (other than a holistic practitioner) anywhere who would be willing to diagnose you with a legitimate disease. Today, you're still going to have to look for someone knowledgeable, and it can be hit and miss (as my experience shows, see chapter 5: Diagnosis). However, many diagnostic tests are available to physicians to pinpoint the cause of the symptoms. The key is to look for a physician who is knowledgeable about the disease. An endocrinologist is usually knowledgeable about hypoglycemic disorders. However, my son's pediatrician also turned out to be very knowledgeable. The key could be to ask your doctor about the Hyperglucidic Breakfast Test; if he knows what it is and he's willing to perform one, it could be that you've met a physician who is willing to take this condition seriously.

References

Larueachagiotis, C., Poussard, A. & Louissylvestre, A. P. (1990). Does Alcohol Promote Reactive Hypoglycemia? *Physiology & Behavior*, 819-823.

Chapter 3: What is Reactive Hypoglycemia?

Reactive hypoglycemia, also known as Postprandial Reactive Hypoglycemia (PRH) in the medical establishment, is a term used to describe the hypoglycemia that occurs 2-4 hours after a meal (usually, a meal high in carbohydrates).

- *Postprandial* = symptoms occur after meals (post "after" + Latin prandium "luncheon")
- *Reactive* = symptoms that occur as a response to food intake
- *Hypoglycemia* = low blood sugar

Simply put, reactive hypoglycemia happens like this: you consume a meal that is typically high in carbs and simple sugars, say, a Big Mac, fries and a Coke or a turkey sandwich on white bread, potato chips and a cola. Your body freaks out at the high sugar load now existing in your blood from all this high-carb food and your pancreas produces too much insulin to try and compensate and bring your blood sugar down. So much insulin, in fact, that the other blood sugar regulators—glucagon and epinephrine—can't cope with the high sugar load in your bloodstream. The result from this imbalance is reactive hypoglycemia—low blood sugar—which causes you to become irritable and lethargic.

If you don't act on your body's signal that you need to eat something, you might get shakes, shivers, chills, and heart palpitations at around the 3 hour mark after eating, or if the Twinkie defense is to be believed, you might become aggressive, violent, or exhibit other kinds of personality disorders (now you know why you told your boss he's an ass at that 11:00 a.m. meeting). Of course, not all reactive hypoglycemics respond to their low blood sugar by buying a gun and shooting the San Francisco Supervisor, but many of us are plagued by an elusive condition that can cause symptoms of stress, depression, mood swings, and PMS-like symptoms.

In experiments on rodents, alcohol and oral glucose combined was shown to trigger reactive hypoglycemia. When combined with stress, the reactive hypoglycemia response worsened (Larueachagiotis et. al 1990).

At first, researchers thought reactive hypoglycemia was connected to diabetes; while diabetics suffer from too little insulin, reactive hypoglycemic exhibit symptoms which seem to suggest they have too much insulin (in fact, when I describe what I have to friends, I often find myself saying I have the opposite of diabetes). The symptoms that reactive hypoglycemics experience with food-induced low blood sugar are indistinguishable from a diabetic experiencing insulin-induced low blood sugar. Simply put, when reactive hypoglycemics eat a carb-heavy meal, they experience an unpleasant reaction usually around two hours after the meal, as their blood sugar drops. Symptoms can be wide and varied, and include:

- Anxiety

- Apathy

- Belligerence

- Blurred vision

- Depression

- Difficulty in thinking

- Dizziness

- Faintness

- Feeling unable to perform complex tasks, like driving

- Hunger

- Irritability

- Lethargy

- Nightmares

- Palpitations

- Personality change

- Rage

- Seizures (blood sugar levels have to be extremely low for this to occur)

- Sleeplessness

- Slurred speech

- Stomach upsets

- Sweating

- Tingling

- Tremors

- Un-coordination (appearing drunk)

- Weakness

You may have just some of the above symptoms. Rarely, reactive hypoglycemia will present itself as an odd set of symptoms that seemingly has no relation to hypoglycemia, or any of the more common symptoms listed above. For instance, in one study, an arthritic patient reported experiencing pain in his hip after sugary meals. Switching to a low carb diet decreased the patient's pain significantly (Lev-Ran, A. & Anderson, R. (1981)

The key is figuring out if your symptoms are occurring after a meal, and if the symptoms are being caused by low blood sugar. One way to determine this is to keep a food diary, noting when your symptoms are occurring. If your symptoms tend to occur 2-4 hours after you ingest high carbs (including alcohol, French fries, baked potatoes, chips, white bread, white pasta, and sodas) it may be time for further diagnostic tools like the Home Glucose Test to determine your blood sugar levels at the time of the symptoms. This is the topic of the next chapter.

Reference

Lev-Ran A, Anderson RW. The diagnosis of postprandial hypoglycemia. *Diabetes,* 1981, *30,* 996-999.

Chapter 4: Tests for Reactive Hypoglycemia

According to modern researchers, there are really only two ways to accurately diagnose reactive hypoglycemia, the *Hyperglucidic Breakfast Test* or *At Home (Ambulatory) Monitoring*. The Hyperglucidic Breakfast Test is ordered by your doctor, while the At Home Monitoring can be performed by you at home with a simple kit available from your local pharmacy. Other tests, like the Glucose Tolerance Test, are no longer recommended by experts on the subject as a sole tool for diagnosing reactive hypoglycemia; they are included in this chapter because they are sometimes used to assess your condition after a diagnosis of reactive hypoglycemia has been made.

Hyperglucidic Breakfast Test

In 1995, French researcher Jean-Frédéric Brun and colleagues developed a "Hyperglucidic breakfast test" to recreate the type of meal that typically causes reactive hypoglycemia.[13] In this test a patient is given a meal of bread, butter, and jam (a breakfast staple in Europe!) along with a serving of milk and powdered coffee, equivalent to a typical high-carbohydrate symptom inducing meal: 9.1% protein, 27.5% fat, and 63.4% carbohydrates.[14] After consuming this meal, your blood will be drawn at several intervals after the test, which is now considered by many to be the standard in testing for reactive hypoglycemia.

At Home Glucose Test

You can do this yourself, if you are comfortable and familiar with blood glucose monitors, or your physician may ask you to perform the test under his guidance. When symptoms occur (sweating, shakiness, palpitations etc.), you prick your finger with a special lancet, wipe a small speck of blood onto a test strip, and insert the strip into a meter. The whole process takes less than five minutes. After the machine gives you your blood glucose level, you note your blood glucose level in your food diary. A look back at your previous meal should give you an indicator of what foods may be causing your symptoms. You should also consume sugar/carbs (for the purposes of this test, *any* high-sugar/carb food will work: a teaspoon of honey, a few pieces of candy, a soda) after you have taken your blood sugar measurement and note if it alleviates the symptoms.

This is the test that I used to aid in the diagnosis of reactive hypoglycemia. When my symptoms occurred, two hours after breakfast, I struggled with my first-time use of the machine. My hands were sweating like I was on a first date and my feet were cold like blocks of ice. I failed to get a reading of anything other than "Error" onscreen; I became more agitated and symptomatic. About to give up, I called customer support and a representative guided me through the correct test procedure. The machine worked with the control solution included in the kit, but not with a drop of blood from my finger. "Are you experiencing symptoms?" The rep asked. "Yes," I replied, and explained that I was agitated, sweating, freezing, and about to faint. "You need to call your doctor," the rep said. "Your blood sugar is too low to read." I didn't call my doctor (at the time, I had no health insurance); I drank 12 ounces of fruit juice instead, following it up with 4 glucose tabs just in case. Thirty minutes later, I tested my blood sugar again. That time, I got an actual reading: 70 mg/dL, which was at the low end of normal. The lesson I learned from this experience is that I eat or drink at the first sign of symptoms now, in order to keep my blood sugar within normal limits. I have no intention of finding out if another 20 years of ups and downs will eventually lead to diabetes.

> I actually obtained my blood glucose monitor for free. Type *free blood glucose monitor* into Google, and you should find one or two companies offering a no-strings attached blood glucose monitor. Mine came with 10 free test strips.

A drawback with this method is that you may be feeling too sick and frustrated to get this gadget to work properly if your blood sugar is too low. A second drawback is that by the time you experience symptoms, your body may already be compensating for too much insulin, and raising your blood glucose levels—by the time you prick your finger, your blood glucose level may already be above the threshold for a reactive hypoglycemia diagnosis. Still, it remains one of the most inexpensive and reliable ways that you can find out what your blood sugar levels are looking like over time.

Hypoglycemia is defined as a serum glucose level (i.e. blood sugar level) of below 70

The Glucose Tolerance Test (GTT)

The three- or five hour Glucose Tolerance Test is perhaps the most widely used test for the diagnosis of reactive hypoglycemia; it is the one my son's pediatrician recommended for a firm diagnosis *after she already had a strong suspicion that he had the condition.* However, if I had been armed with the information I had today, I would not have put my son through this test. Ten-year-old Leo had to fast for 10 hours (overnight). After waiting an hour for a phlebotomist (that's the person who draws the blood), a blood sample was taken from his arm and he was asked to drink an orange flavored glucose drink at about 9:30 a.m. His blood was drawn five more times over the course of three hours. Leo was a good sport about it, but as any kid will tell you, being stuck with a needle and having your blood drawn six times over the course of three hours doesn't exactly rate as fun.

Leo's results showed a high (180 mg/dL) and low (60 mg/dL) an hour later that is typical of reactive hypoglycemia. His hypoglycemia was accompanied by the typical kinds of symptoms he experienced occasionally—cold feet and hands, feeling sick to his stomach, moodiness and general malaise. Thankfully his blood sugar didn't dip so low at that time to precipitate another seizure.

Although the GTT is the most widely used test, the high number of false positives—where patients experience reactive hypoglycemia on the test and not in everyday life--also makes it one of the most unreliable tests and researchers think it should not be used as a sole tool for diagnostic purposes.[15]

Leo's positive result on this test was bolstered by a history of seizures, and the fact that on several occasions, orange juice had revived him just seconds before he passed out. Plus he experienced symptoms during the test that were alleviated by drinking juice once the test had finished (I can't tell you how happy that kid was to guzzle down a carton of orange juice after not eating for 18 hours!).

The Breakfast Test

This is not the same thing as a Hyperglucidic Breakfast test. In the Breakfast Test, a person eats a "normal" breakfast (i.e. cereal, tea, and sugar) designed by a hospital's diet department. Many studies have shown that the mixed meal typically served for this test fails to reproduce the reactive hypoglycemia that patients experience at home,[16] perhaps because cereal, tea, and sugar doesn't come close to approximating the large coffee and donuts of the typical American diet.

The hypoglycemic index

This blood test measures the drop in plasma glucose during the hour and a half before the glucose level drops to its nadir (the lowest level.) The measure of the drop, divided by the low point, is called the "hypoglycemic index." This test is no longer used because several researchers have concluded it is not valid for the diagnosis of hypoglycemia.[17]

Chapter 5: Diagnosis

After your doctor has ordered tests to diagnose reactive hypoglycemia, a formal diagnosis of reactive hypoglycemia will be given under the following conditions:

- The possibility of diabetes or prediabetes as a factor is ruled out. This is important because the glucose intolerance experienced by many pre-diabetic and early-stage patients can look remarkably similar to reactive hypoglycemia. The chart on the following page illustrates how glucose intolerance symptoms can mimic those of reactive hypoglycemia; the reactive hypoglycemic patient will most likely see a sharp drop at the 2-3 hour mark, whereas the patient with glucose intolerance might see a longer amount of time before a blood sugar drop. Also, the glucose intolerant patient might see hyperglycemia (glucose levels that are too high, above 180 mg/dL) as well as hypoglycemia.

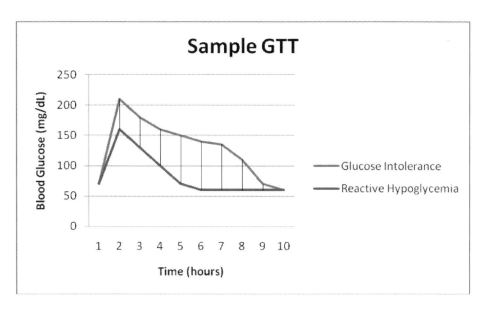

Sample GTT

Blood Glucose (mg/dL)

Glucose Intolerance
Reactive Hypoglycemia

Time (hours)

- Mental illness will be ruled out by your physician (this could be slightly problematic, considering the history of physicians misdiagnosing reactive hypoglycemia, but considering the relatively high rate of mental illness, it is a necessary evil). However, if your doctor tells you that your symptoms are due to "stress," and this diagnosis doesn't feel right—don't take no for an answer—insist on a Hyperglucidic Breakfast Test, support for ambulatory testing, or find another doctor!

- Even though the Hyperglucidic Breakfast Test or an at-home glucose testing kit has been used to determine your glucose levels, your doctor may at this point order further testing (including a GTT for diagnostic purposes).

If your glucose level is 50 mg/dl or higher (still very low)[18], your doctor will consider the "Whipple Triad"; if you can answer yes to the following three questions you are most likely to be diagnosed with reactive hypoglycemia.

1. Do you have physical symptoms typical of hypoglycemia?

2. Do you also have low plasma glucose (as shown by the Hyperglucidic Breakfast Test)?

3. Do your physical symptoms disappear when your glucose levels return to normal?

The answer to all three questions must be yes in order for a diagnosis of reactive hypoglycemia.[19]

Unfortunately, obtaining a diagnosis isn't as easy as it sounds. As discussed at the beginning of this book, people with reactive hypoglycemia have suffered from misdiagnosis and ignorance about the disorder for decades. Even though modern research has identified all of the causes of reactive hypoglycemia, many physicians are not up to date with the current research, or for other reasons don't recognize reactive hypoglycemia as a real disease.

My own personal experience with this mentality was when I asked my current doctor about my symptoms and was told it was due to stress (actually, "current doctor" is somewhat of a misnomer—after his "diagnosis," I have no intention of going back.

The Doctor's Visit

I wouldn't have made an appointment with my physician if I hadn't been concerned that, considering both my son Leo and I had the same disorder, that we might have an underlying condition. A missing liver enzyme perhaps, or some other hereditary disorder.

My idea was that if the doctor could pinpoint a cause, the doctor might be able to solve our problem with a simple supplement or the like, instead of a very restrictive diet. At the time, I didn't know too much about reactive hypoglycemia, just what I had read on the internet, which wasn't much. The information that I did read was confusing and sometimes unhelpful: to eat soup or to not eat soup? Avoid carbs? Eat a balanced diet? Assume I have prediabetes? See an acupuncturist? Move to a thin atmosphere like Denver? Eat rambling powder, as suggested by a practitioner of Chinese Medicine? Get tested for diabetes?

I thought I was making a good choice when I specifically chose an Internal Medicine doctor from my health plan, thinking that an "expert" in puzzling, chronic problems would be my best choice (an internal medicine doctor is sometimes called "the doctor's doctor" because of their expertise in pinpointing conditions with a myriad of symptoms).

It turns out that doctors—even internal medicine doctors— are only human.

The doctor, I'll call him Dr. Brown, listened as I explained that my son and I had the same symptoms, that I had monitored my blood sugar and it appeared I might have reactive hypoglycemia. I also told him about how my son had recently been diagnosed by his pediatrician. I asked him if I should be concerned about any hereditary disorders.

He did a quick physical examination and asked me if I felt stressed. Puzzled, I noticed that my hands were sweaty. "My hands sweat when my blood sugar dips" I said. *Yes, of course I'm stressed. Wouldn't you be if you'd spent the last year or so having unexplained panic spells, with freezing limbs, flu-like symptoms, and disturbed sleep?*

He nodded, left the room, and returned with a sheet of paper. He handed it to me and asked me if any of the items pertained to me. The top of the sheet said "Signs of Depression" and included questions like "Are you having difficulty sleeping?" Of *course* I was having trouble sleeping. My blood glucose would drop in the middle of the night, and I would have a nightmare—my body's way of dealing with the stressors of hypoglycemia. I would wake up at 4 a.m. frequently, and not be able to get to sleep again until I ate. "Do you have thoughts of worthlessness?" "I'm not depressed," I said. "I feel fine, except after I eat certain foods like potatoes or lasagna…" He nodded thoughtfully, told me I needed to lose weight because I was at risk for diabetes. I was five pounds overweight. *At risk for diabetes?* I recalled that I had looked on the internet for signs of diabetes when my symptoms first occurred, and I didn't seem to fit the profile.

He handed me a sheet of paper.

Risk factors for diabetes

Over 45

Gestational Diabetes (during pregnancy)

Overweight

Family history of diabetes

Giving birth to a baby weighing more than 9 pounds

HDL cholesterol under 35

High blood levels of triglycerides (250 mg/dL or more)

High blood pressure (greater than or equal to 140/90 mmHg)

Impaired glucose tolerance

Low activity level

Poor diet

I was 41 when symptoms got really bad (although I suspect I've been reactive hypoglycemic my whole life). I hadn't had diabetes during any of my pregnancies, and although I was 5 pounds overweight, I was active, exercising almost every day, including Tae Kwon Do, swimming, and biking. I had no family history of diabetes, although my first son weighted more than 9 pounds. My latest blood test revealed my HDL and triglycerides were the exact *opposite* of what one would expect to see in a diabetic patient, and my diet was vegetarian. I had perhaps 20% of the symptoms on that sheet of paper, and if the current American epidemic of obesity, junk food and sedentary lifestyle is to be measure against the "Diabetes Risk" fact sheet, I was right up there with 90% of the US population.

He handed me another sheet, this time titled "Diabetes Symptoms." I opened and closed my mouth like a fish, unable to formulate the words; *you have to be kidding me, right? Were you even listening?* "Hypoglycemia is one of the first symptoms of pre-diabetes," he said. "Lose weight, and exercise more. Avoid carbs and root vegetables like potatoes and carrots. Come back for a check-up in six months."

> *Diabetes Symptoms:*
> **Frequent Bathroom Trips**
> **Unquenchable Thirst**
> **Fatigue/Weakness**
> **Tingling in hands, legs, or feet**

I left the doctor's office in a fog, and read the "Diabetes Symptoms" sheet in the car. I had the "tingling" in my hands and feet, but only 2 hours after I ate.

I felt like I'd just been duped by a used car salesman trying to make a quick buck: that's the only way I can explain how I felt when I went in so certain with my diagnosis, but coming away with something completely different than when I went in. Diabetes? I wondered. I hadn't even considered it. Considering my son had reactive hypoglycemia, I'd assumed the doctor would be interested in why mother and son were suffering from this seemingly rare disorder, and order a test or two to find out what was genetically wrong. Instead, I came away with a couple of informational sheets on diabetes and depression—the patient's equivalent of a pacifier. The question I asked myself all day was, *why didn't he listen to me?*

Chapter 6: Causes

Reactive hypoglycemia occurs when the body's glucose regulatory system fails to work properly. It's basically where something is amiss in the regulatory system that controls how much glucose is coming in to your system, and how much is going out.[20] The complex cornucopia of regulatory hormones that keep blood sugar levels normal can be disturbed by many things including epinephrine, insulin, glucagon, cortisol, and growth hormone imbalances.[21]

It used to be that doctors didn't know the cause of reactive hypoglycemia, but most of the underlying physiological causes are now known; it is not correct any more to state that reactive hypoglycemia is a disease of unknown cause. It may be hard to track it down, but there's always a cause because reactive hypoglycemia is a set of symptoms, not a disease. Here are some of the more common causes and a few of the rarer ones) of reactive hypoglycemia.

Common Causes

Giftedness

I don't usually tell people that my son, Leo is academically gifted (i.e. he has a high IQ), for risk of sounding boorish. My close friends and family know, but it isn't the kind of thing I'll bring up in general conversation, let alone post in a blog. However, it looks like Leo's giftedness may be the reason he's reactive hypoglycemic.

For years I thought Leo (now ten years old) had cyclothymia (a mild form of bipolar disorder). He would have mood swings and highs reminiscent of my mother's menopause: doors would slam, dishes would smash against the kitchen wall, and then an hour later, Leo would (puzzlingly) make tea for me, give me a hug, and apologize in the sweetest way you could imagine for being a "toad." At the time, I didn't notice that his mood improved after a snack.

Sometimes he would come home from school and go to bed for a two hour nap. I knew better than to disturb him—it was either let him sleep or put up with a miserable, grumpy Leo.

Leo's schoolwork was haphazard—sometimes brilliant, other times nothing but scrawl and misspellings. His teachers were as puzzled as I was. Another thing that didn't make sense: Leo would crave sweets and carbs so much that he would often raid the kitchen late at night for cookies, chips, and crackers (I no longer keep those items in the house!)

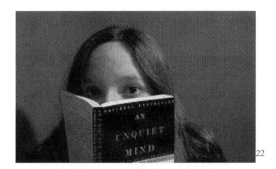

While Leo seemed to fit the definition of bipolar, his puzzling seizures (two Grand mals) didn't quite fit the profile. Neither did his spells of feeling nauseous and looking pasty-faced before he passed out. After he was diagnosed with reactive hypoglycemia, the pieces of the puzzle fell into place. However, we wanted to know the cause. Wouldn't any parent?

I may have found my answer in a book by James Webb, called *Misdiagnosis and Dual Diagnosis of Gifted Children*. About six percent of highly-gifted children, says Webb, suffer from reactive hypoglycemia. The children who fall into this category are usually slender and exhibit intense behavior. Leo is definitely intense, and *very slim*. Why is reactive hypoglycemia seen in these children? As the brain runs on glucose alone, it's thought that highly gifted, energetic children simply use up available brain fuel quickly.

If your child is a good student but exhibits puzzling mood swings, especially in the late morning or late afternoon, reactive hypoglycemia could be the cause.

Helicobacter Pylori Infection

A common stomach bacterium can lead to reactive hypoglycemia, according to current research.[23] If you have other symptoms such as bloating or nausea, a breath test from your doctor can rule of the presence of this bacterium.

Insulin, Epinephrine, and Glucagon Sensitivities & Deficiencies

Many hormones are interdependent, and it isn't an easy task for researchers (or your physician) to pin down the exact culprit. A 1971 study[24] suggested that an exaggerated insulin response could be the major cause of reactive hypoglycemic. Due to overlapping symptoms, an exaggerated insulin response is similar to epinephrine sensitivity. However an exaggerated insulin response will produce a low blood sugar level, while the epinephrine sensitivity will not. When a reactive hypoglycemic eats a meal high in carbs, the body responds by producing a large shot of insulin, resulting in insulinemia, an abnormal concentration of insulin in the blood. This high concentration of insulin results in the unpleasant side effects of hypoglycemia, and will often subside within a short time period until enough epinephrine is released to balance the insulin. The body's natural reaction to this influx of insulin is to balance the insulin with compensatory epinephrine. This is where it gets complicated: individuals with sensitivity to epinephrine will have symptoms of hypoglycemia–shakes, anxiety, sweats etc. Additionally, stress causes *more* epinephrine to be released, so being anxious about the pounding heart, palpitations and other unpleasant side effects of epinephrine in epinephrine sensitive individuals will lead to more epinephrine being released, and more anxiety. How to decide if epinephrine sensitivity or insulinemia might apply to you? There's no real way of being sure other than to undergo medical tests. However, you can get an idea if like me, you discover you are sensitive to epinephrine in the dentist chair (some anesthetics contain epinephrine). Monitoring my blood sugar helped me to determine that epinephrine alone was not the culprit. As of time of writing, Leo and I are still searching for the cause of our reactive hypoglycemia, and we haven't ruled out some type of hereditary insulinemia. Closely related to an exaggerated insulin response is an exaggerated response of glucagon-like-peptide-1 (GLP-1), which will also cause an increase in insulin[25] and a defect in glucagon. These types of diagnosis can only be received with lab tests.

Alimentary hypoglycemia

If you have had a total or partial gastroectomy (i.e. you've had gastric bypass surgery) and you are experiencing reactive hypoglycemia with nausea, a feeling of fullness, weakness and heart palpitations, you could be suffering from dumping syndrome, where the stomach empties too fast into the small intestine.

Body Type

Reactive hypoglycemia often occurs in three specific types of people (although it is not limited to these people):

- Very lean people[26]

- People who have lost a lot of weight through slimming[27]

- Women with a moderately overweight (not obese) in their lower body. Women from this group often report "carb cravings" along with late morning reactive hypoglycemia, and so munch carb-loaded snacks and continue to gain weight.[28]

Diet

Not surprisingly, a poor diet is a contributing factor to reactive hypoglycemia. Well-conducted studies on this subject are lacking, but some studies indicate that a low fat, high carb diet contributes to reactive hypoglycemia.[29] Internist Richard Podell[30] states that 40% of his patients with sugar-related problems improve after they start an anti-hypoglycemic diet: one that is free of simple carbs like white bread and pasta, and is sugar, caffeine and alcohol restricted. Also, people on a calorie restricted diet may also be at risk, especially when eating primarily high-carb foods. Other factors that may contribute to the disease include alcohol (one experiment showed that the equivalent of three gin and tonics can cause reactive hypoglycemia[31]) and there is also a possibility that a calcium deficiency in the diet may be a cause.[32]

Prediabetes

Prediabetes is rarely mentioned as a possible cause of reactive hypoglycemia. However, hypoglycemia, reactive hypoglycemia, and glucose tolerance are closely related and can cause similar symptoms. Typically, a prediabetic patient will not only have hypoglycemia but they will also have hyperglycemia, or high blood sugar.[33] It's worth considering prediabetes as a possible cause for what you think is reactive hypoglycemia if you have risk factors for diabetes (see the "risk factors for diabetes" list in the previous chapter).

Insulinoma

Insulinoma is a rare (4 cases per 1 million person-years[34]) liver tumor that requires a 48 to 72 hour fasting test to diagnose.[35] Insulinomas are not easy to diagnose, and many patients in the past were misdiagnosed with a psychiatric illnesses or a seizure disorder before this disease was recognized,[36] perhaps because a patient with insulinoma may appear aggressive and confused.[37] Your doctor may order a fasting test if your symptoms are severe and do not respond to dietary changes.[38] However, do the extreme rarity of this disease, if you have reactive hypoglycemia it is highly unlikely that insulinoma is the cause of your symptoms.

Galactosemia and Hereditary Fructose Intolerance

Both very rare disorders, people with these diseases will typically have an enlarged liver, be jaundiced, and vomit after meals[39], as well as experiencing reactive hypoglycemia.

Renal glycosuria

If increased insulin isn't present, there is a possibility of renal glycosuria, a rare disorder where glucose is excreted in the urine.

High insulin sensitivity

Thought to be a major cause of reactive hypoglycemia, it is not thought that high insulin sensitivity by itself causes hypoglycemia, rather it works with other factors (i.e. abnormally low glucagon production) to produce reactive hypoglycemia.[40]

This is not an exhaustive list: abnormalities of other counter regulatory hormones may exist in this disease, and practically nothing is known about them.[41]

Yeast Infections

The systemic kind, that is —not the usual yeast infections that women suffer from.

In January of 2010, my health plummeted downhill. I thought I had my reactive hypoglycemia under control, and then things suddenly went to pot. The list of foods I was able to eat with experiencing a severe hypoglycemic episode (blood glucose levels below 40 mg/dL) dwindled to apples and walnuts. By July, I was so ill I was unable to walk up a flight of stairs. All of the regular doctors said there was nothing they could do for me. "Gastroenteritis," said one. "A virus," said another.

I don't quite remember why I went to see a Naturopathic physician. I'm pretty sure it was an act of desperation. After all, I was down to eating apples and walnuts. I was lactose intolerant, gluten intolerant, and...well, food intolerant. If I ate anything at all, an hour or two later my blood sugar would crash horribly to around 20-30 mg/dL. I was spending more and more days in bed, not wanting to eat, depressed and unable to face the world. To make matters worse, even though I didn't want to eat, I had to eat: every hour and a half. Otherwise, I slipped into a semi-coma. I had blackout periods that were extremely scary for my family.

The first thing my naturopath did was to test me for food allergies. The test came back, surprisingly, negative (except for a mild allergy to eggs). This was a bit of a puzzle, as it seemed I reacted to everything! He then suggested I get an Adrenal Stress Index test. When this test came back, it indicated my cortisol was four times higher than normal. A normal 8 a.m. reading was 6 to 23 mcg/dL: mine was 103 mcg/dL.

What causes high cortisol levels? There are many possible causes including depression, stress, and Cushing's disease. But mine was caused by nocturnal hypoglycemia. Essentially, my blood sugar would drop in the middle of the night and my body would go into a stress induced panic attack, causing nightmares, restless sleep, and those high cortisol levels.

The final piece of the puzzle was a questionnaire from my doctor and a few educated guesses of what the cause might be. My medical history revealed I'd had a strong reaction to an antibiotic a year previously.

His diagnosis? A systemic yeast infection. The antibiotics killed all of the bacteria in my gut, causing the yeast to become rampant, enter my bloodstream and infect my organs. Additionally, the yeast had eaten through my lower intestine, allowing particles of undigested food to swim around in my bloodstream. No wonder I felt sick. My blood was 10 percent walnuts and apples. In a healthy person, a yeast infection could be a major problem. In someone with reactive hypoglycemia, the problem could have been deadly. My gut was unable to absorb enough nutrients to raise my blood sugar so just a tiny drop in glucose levels was critical for me.

Thankfully, I fully recovered from the illness with no long term side effects. It takes 3-4 months to recover from a systemic yeast infection. I took huge doses of probiotics and B12 and also took Seriphos (to lower Cortisol levels) and Hawthorn berry (to help with the cortisol-induced heart palpitations).

If you are reactive hypoglycemic , if it seems severe and sometime in the distant past you took antibiotics, take a trip to a natural foods store and purchase a quality probiotic.

And as a side note: If you have reactive hypoglycemia and you wake up in the morning feeling anxious, go to a naturpoath for an adrenal stress index. It's one more piece of the puzzle that could lead you to a cure.

Celiac Disease / Wheat and Gluten Allergies

As part of my journey with discovering what exactly was causing my reactive hypoglycemia, I received a comment from blogger Erica Douglas who suggested that my symptoms might be caused by celiac disease. Celiac disease is a fairly common autoimmune disease where the small intestine's lining is damaged from gluten and other proteins in wheat, barley, and rye.

As I begun to look into the disease, I noticed many similarities with the symptoms of reactive hypoglycemia. However, there were a few off and on symptoms that both I and my son had which weren't explained by reactive hypoglycemia alone: namely, gas, bloating, diarrhea, and lactose intolerance. As we don't have health insurance, a test was out of the question (the test would have cost a minimum of six hundred dollars) so we did a little experiment and cut all gluten products out of our diet in the summer of 2010. The result was nothing short of miraculous for my son, who no longer passes gas every time he sits down. We used to joke about his farts, thinking they were a normal part of growing up or perhaps a result of us eating too many starchy, fiber-filled foods on our vegan diet. Now we realize they were due to ingesting gluten.

Many celiac patients experience hypoglycemia as a result of celiac disease. With celiac, simple carbs are absorbed through the stomach lining and more complex carbs, which should be absorbed in the small intestine, aren't absorbed at all. The result is a complex pattern of apparent reactive hypoglycemia.

Like reactive hypoglycemia, celiac disease can have an array of hard to diagnose symptoms:

- Abdominal cramping/bloating

- Feet (Reduced fat padding)

- Abdominal distentionFlatus (Passing gas)

- Acidosis

- Gluten ataxia

- Appetite (Increased to the point of craving)

- Mouth sores or cracks in the corners

- Back pain (Such as a result of collapsed lumbar vertebrae)

- Muscle cramping (Especially in the hands and legs)

- Constipation

- Night blindness

- Decreased ability to clot blood

- Skin (Very dry)

- Dehydration

- Stools (Loose? Hard? Small? Large? Foul smelling? Floating? Clay, Light tan or Gray-colored? Highly rancid? Frothy?)

- Diarrhea

- Tongue (Smooth or geographic - looks like different continents)

- Edema

- Tooth enamel defects

- Electrolyte depletion

- Weakness

- Energy loss

- Weight loss

- Fatigue

If you have reactive hypoglycemia and you haven't yet found the cause, consider celiac disease as a potential culprit, especially if you also experience any of the symptoms of celiac. For more information about celiac disease, you can visit CSA Celiacs website at www.csaceliacs.org.

Chapter 7: Treatment Options

DIET

In one study in the mid-1980s, researchers gave eight subjects suspected of having reactive hypoglycemia a euglycemic (blood sugar friendly) diet. Symptoms (including depression) disappeared on the euglycemic diet, but when the subjects returned to their previous junk food diets, all experienced reactive hypoglycemia again. The researchers concluded that a diet free of refined sugar and caffeine helps alleviate depression, anxiety, and fatigue in people with reactive hypoglycemia.[42]

However, this was a tiny study; if only it were as easy as not drinking coffee and avoiding sugar. Everyone's body is different, and finding the right diet for reactive hypoglycemia can be frustrating. There is no "magic diet" – it's really a case of trial and error. All diets for reactive hypoglycemia recommend the elimination of caffeine and sugars (fructose is okay in some), the reduction of refined carbs, and state that that those vegetables with a low glycemic index can be eaten often.

Supplements like flax seed, nutritional yeast flakes, vitamins, calcium supplements, lipoic acid, *Gymnema sylvestre,* 5-HTTP, St. John's Wort, and garlic have been proposed by some to ameliorate the symptoms of reactive hypoglycemia,[43] and they certainly can't hurt.

The diet recommended by Seale Harris was the elimination of all fresh fruits, whole grains, and legumes with the majority of calories coming from fatty animal products. Later diets (including the Atkins) built upon this and encouraged a high-protein, low-carb intake (including the reduction of starchy vegetables and fruit), mega doses of vitamins. In addition, there were a few quirky diets that recommended receiving full spectrum light, avoiding microwave ovens, and only eating raw milk and fertile eggs.

The glycemic index ranks carbohydrates according to their effect on blood sugar levels. Although the glycemic index can be helpful in sorting out which foods to avoid and which to favor, it shouldn't be relied upon as the only source of information about diet.

The Paavo Airola diet is low in animal products and high in whole grains, nuts seeds, legumes, vegetables and fruit.[44] It is this diet that worked for me, so most of this chapter is based around that premise.

Whatever diet you choose, a low-carb diet and frequent small split meals should be the first treatment for reactive hypoglycemia.[45] Adding two small meals, one mid-morning and one mid-afternoon, should be the first step.[46] I also found that eating a slice of Ezekiel 4:9

with 2 tablespoons of peanut butter immediately before bed helps my blood glucose stabilize overnight. I've tried various other foods: handfuls of peanuts, a low-carb, high-protein snack bar, high-protein, low carb raisin-bread, but nothing works for me like the Ezekiel 4:9 no-wheat bread. A high-fiber, restricted-simple sugar diet full of fruits and vegetables is a must. In other words, skip the Big Mac and have a Southwestern Salad instead. Load on all the veggies at Subway, choose the wholewheat bread and skip the chips and soda (yes, even the baked chips). Here are some tips to follow when creating your new diet:

Tip #1: Eat Carbohydrates

Your body needs carbs to regulate blood sugar. You may have already encountered some websites that recommend things like "55% of energy as carbohydrate" in a diet or "try a low carb, high protein diet" or "less than x grams of simple carbohydrate daily." That's easy for a dietician to plan, but who really has time to plan meals like that? Additionally, do you follow the high carb, low protein diet advocated by some, or the low GI diet? As well as all this information being confusing, in the meantime, your blood sugar is up and down like a yoyo, and who feels like cooking then? The simple answer is to follow a few easy steps, and gradually make changes in your diet.

Tip #2: Swap white bread and noodles for whole grains.

There's no doubt about it, there are going to be those times you don't feel like cooking, and you reach for something simple, like a sandwich or a burger in a bun. That's why it's important to replace the products you normally buy with their whole grain alternatives (when you reach in freezer and grab a wholewheat bun and a bean burger, it's impossible to feel guilt!). Complex carbohydrates like whole grain crackers, bagels, and cereal deliver glucose over a longer period of time, resulting in a slower sugar response.

Tip #3: Choose cereals carefully

Shop in a health food store if you can, because you are more likely to find "hidden" ingredients in name brand cereal like High Fructose Corn Syrup or Sugar. Did you know that the first ingredient in Apple Jacks is sugar? I only found that out after my son, Leo, consumed a large bowl and hours later was in a bad mood thanks to a blood sugar drop. Look for low-carb, no sugar cereals like Kamut Flakes or Kashi Whole Grain Puffs. Ezekiel 4:9 bread is Low GI, and full of protein. You can use that instead of regular bread, but you can try another (no sugar) whole grain product.

Tip #4: Drink water or non-caffeinated tea instead of soda

There is some research to suggest that some artificial sweeteners may produce an insulin response,[47] so they are best avoided, especially considering many soft drinks also contain caffeine! Buy spritzer water or lime-flavored sparkling water. I've tried just about every herbal tea in the book, and I settled on one that actually tasted good (like hot lemonade): Lemon Mate. You *may* be able to tolerate caffeine; I learned to restrict coffee to one, very small cup in the morning. Any more than that precipitates a blood sugar crash for me.

Tip #5: Eat every two hours

Only you can determine how often you need to eat (that's why it's a good idea to check your blood sugar using a home blood glucose monitoring device and make sure you eat before your blood sugar gets a chance to dip below 70 mg/dL), but the two hour rule works for most people to avoid a crash. That equates to about eight meals a day, starting at 8 a.m. and finishing at 10 p.m. It's important to take the portion of food that you would normally eat for a meal, and split it into two (or one third and two thirds). For example, I eat the cereal at 8 and the toast at 10. I do the same for lunch, and divide what I would normally eat into two meals (i.e. I eat the sandwich and fruit at noon and the soup at 2).

Tip #6: Read Your Labels

I shop at a local health food store, because I became so frustrated at buying products at local grocery stores. Food manufacturers sneak sugar and High Fructose Corn Syrup into everything! For example, I bought home two jars of Planter's Dry Roasted Peanuts, and was dismayed to find out later on that they put sugar on them as a coating. Even small amounts of sugar spike my blood sugar and cause a crash so I absolutely have to avoid it if I am to maintain and even blood sugar level. I had a similar problem buying yogurt, bread, and just about every product you can think of. Organic products and vegan products (i.e. soy yogurt instead of regular) tend to be sweetened with evaporated cane syrup, which does not cause blood sugar spikes like sugar and high fructose corn syrup.

Tip #7: Learn to Love Fruit and Veggies

It took some getting used to, but we purged our cupboards of snack foods except for whole grain crackers, vegan cream cheese, and fruits/veggies. We eat stir fries, soups, salads, vegan chili, and other dishes bursting with vegetables. A diet rich in fruits and vegetables is a must to maintain blood sugar levels.

Tip #8: Drink and Eat Before You Exercise

Exercise lowers your blood sugar, which is great for diabetics, but not so great for the reactive hypoglycemic. I have to drink fruit juice and eat half an energy bar before I exercise, and fruit juice plus the other half of the bar afterward, otherwise I cannot exercise without feeling sick.

Tip #9: What to do if Your Blood Sugar Drops.

When blood glucose drops, high carb foods can bring it back up to normal; at the first sign of low blood sugar (shakes, sweaty hands, churning stomach or another symptom which may be specific to you), you *must* eat a meal or a snack. Diabetics will often consume sugar, candy, or soda to raise blood sugar quickly. This is a *bad idea* for reactive hypoglycemics and is unnecessary. If you learn to eat at the first sign of symptoms, you will ward off a hypoglycemic attack. In an emergency, choose glucose tablets (available in the diabetic section of your local pharmacy) followed by nuts or a wholegrain bagel, or fruit juice over candy or cola, which will quickly spike your blood sugar and encourage it to fall rapidly.

Tip #10: Carry a Snack Everywhere You Go

Packs of nuts, a piece of fruit, or a healthy drink (i.e. a small carton of apple juice). Carry something so that at the first sign of something amiss – you have something to eat.

Tip #11: Keep a Jar of Pectin or Guar Gum in Your Cupboard and Use it as a Food Additive.

Pectin (a fiber found in apples, citrus fruits, grapes, berries, and bran) and guar (used as a thickening agent in many products like yogurt and sauces) have been shown to improve reactive hypoglycemia.[48]

Tip #12: Keep a Food Diary

Keeping a food diary can be the first step toward controlling your reactive hypoglycemia. If you see a dietician, make sure you take your notes with you, so that the dietician can better design a diet for you. There are so many causes for reactive hypoglycemia; there is no "miracle diet" that will work for everyone. It took me a month of trial and error to find a balance for my condition. I noted which foods caused my blood sugar to crash and I avoided them completely, eating only those things I knew for certain would not cause my symptoms to appear. I went on a severe carb and calorie restricted diet (I was desperate to stop my symptoms). This meant that for the first month, my family wasn't too fussed about being served soup and salad for dinner, every night. We had plenty of "variation": lentil soup and Caesar salad, vegetable soup and garden salad, minestrone (whole wheat macaroni) and Mandarin orange salad. And yes, it was boring, but worth it because I didn't get sick. Lunches and breakfasts were made from a few basic ingredients: Quorn (a chicken substitute), vegetables and fruits, wholegrain products, Vegenaise, and a handful of no-sugar, unrefined, no animal-product items.

My blood sugar tanked one day for no good reason at all. I micro-studied my diet for the next few days to try and identify the culprit. I failed and thought it was just a "blip"-- one of those blood sugar moments that has no cause. I was wrong: I found my solution one morning in my decaf coffee cup.

I gave up drinking caffeine some time ago although I drink 4-5 cups of decaf per day. Along with my health eating regime, which includes lots of fruits and veggies, my blood sugar stabilized but one week in the Fall of 2010, I felt sick and ill in the afternoons. My fingers were ice cold and I knew it was blood sugar. I blamed stress, or thought I'd forgotten a supplement or two (a probiotics, an adrenal supplement or caprylate). I hadn't.

One morning, I went to make my third cup of Seattle's Best Organic Decaf Coffee. I read the package as I waited for the coffee to brew and realized it was full caffeine and not decaf. Unknown to me, I had been consuming caffeinated coffee all week, since grocery shopping on Monday. I had my answers...caffeine was tanking my blood sugar.

Of course, I wasn't about to take my own word for it and pronounce to the world that caffeine tanks your blood sugar and decaf is good for you. So I did a little research. I didn't have to go very far. A CBS new story highlighted a recent study on diabetes sufferers (you can find the link to the article in the Further Reading section of this book). The conclusion of the study was that there's something in decaf coffee that helps to control blood sugar and there's something in caffeine that stops your body from regulating sugar properly. That almost worth repeating: it isn't enough to just not drink caffeinated coffee if you have problems with regulating blood sugar – you should start drinking decaf coffee instead.

Pharmaceutical Solutions

If diet does not improve your symptoms, it could be time to approach your doctor about medicines to help alleviate your symptoms. There are several drugs available to treat reactive hypoglycemia that does not respond to diet therapy. Your doctor might prescribe one of the following:

Acarbose (i.e. Precose by Bayer Pharmaceuticals). An anti-diabetic drug that stops the full digestion of carbohydrates.

Atropine. An anticholinergic drug that blocks the effects of the neurotransmitter acetylcholine. Blocking this brain chemical can slow down the rate of stomach emptying, and help prevent hypoglycemia from occurring.

Biguanides. A drug that is normally used to *lower* blood sugar concentrations in diabetes has been shown to be effective with the treatment of reactive hypoglycemia.

Calcium gluconate. A mineral supplement used to treat calcium deficiencies.

Chromium supplement. A mineral supplement used to treat chromium deficiencies.

Diazoxide. Works to prevent hypoglycemia by inhibiting the release of insulin from the pancreas. Usually employed only in severe cases of reactive hypoglycemia.

Diltiazem. A calcium channel blocker. Usually prescribed to slow heart rate, it's been shown to help prevent hypoglycemic attacks.

Intestinal alpha-glucosidase inhibitors. Like *acarbose*, this is an anti-diabetic drug that stops the full digestion of carbohydrates.

Metformin. The most commonly prescribed anti-diabetes drug (usually prescribed for diabetic patients who are obese with insulin resistance), *metformin* has been shown to be useful in treating reactive hypoglycemia in combination with diet.

Miglitol. An oral anti-diabetic drug that inhibits the body's ability to turn complex carbohydrates into glucose.

Nicardipine. A calcium antagonist. Has been shown in limited studies to have some use in fighting reactive hypoglycemia.

Nifedipine. A calcium blocker, also shown in a few small studies to have some use against reactive hypoglycemia.

Phenytoin. Usually prescribed to treat epilepsy, this drug has been shown to improve symptoms of reactive hypoglycemia.

Pioglitazone An exciting piece of research came out of Japan in October of 2009 and was published in a Japanese Clinical Neurology journal called Rinnsho Shinkeigaku.[49] The case study was of a nondiabetic, 20-year-old woman with myotonic dystrophy (an inherited, degenerative disorder) who suffered from reactive hypoglycemia. Her blood glucose level went down to 57 mg/dl at the 120 minute mark of an Oral Glucose Tolerance Test and she was diagnosed with reactive hypoglcyemia. Pioglitazone treatment improved her results on the Oral Glucose Tolerance Test and relieved her symptoms.

Pioglitazone is a drug used for the treatment of type 2 diabetes. It is what is called a "thiazolidinedione antidiabetic;" it lowers blood sugar by making cells more sensitive to insulin. By lowering the body's sensitivity to insulin, pioglitazone also alleviates the major problem for reactive hypoglycemics: an over-reaction to high insulin and the resultant plummeting blood sugar levels.

Should this mean we should all rush out and ask for the drug? Probably not--but it's wonderful that researchers are finally taking this disease seriously and looking for answers. It's important also to note that use of Pioglitazone comes with certain risks, including an increased risk of heart failure. Reactive hypoglycemia comes with a host of unpleasant symptoms, but unlike type 2 diabetes isn't life threatening. It's worth considering whether your symptoms justify an increase in heart failure risk (along with all of the other side effects inherent in taking prescription medication).

Propantheline. A drug that reduces the secretions of some organs in the body. It has been used to prevent hypoglycemic attacks in some cases.

Propranolol. A calcium antagonist.

Somatostatin analogues. One researcher showed that somatostatin slowed the initial rise in blood sugar and delayed the onset of hypoglycemia.[50] However, this drug is diabetogenic (is capable of producing diabetes). Usually prescribed only in severe cases of reactive hypoglycemia that don't respond to other treatment.

Chapter 8: Sample Diets and Suggested Foods.

The following sample diet is an example of what I ate for the first month. There was very little variation on this. I chose different breakfast cereals from the suggested foods list, substituting it on some days for the toast. Each day was a different soup and salad, and I swapped out the Quorn & Chicken stir fry for other vegetable and nutrient rich dishes. This sample diet has no sugar, is high in fiber and nutrients, low fat, and is low on the glycemic index. Recipe suggestions can be found in the companion book to this edition, *The Reactive Hypoglycemia Cookbook*. You'll find more information about that in the References and Further Reading section of this book.

Sample Diet for the first month

Breakfast (8 a.m.)

1 slice of Ezekiel 4:9 plain toast with buttery spread

1 cup homemade, no-sugar pinto beans

Mid-morning snack (10 a.m.)

1 piece of low-sugar fruit (i.e. apple or greenish banana)

Lunch (noon)

Quorn Chik'n stir fry (Quorn, veggies, canola oil, a few spices)

Afternoon snack (2 p.m.)

1 cup apple juice, 4 small wholegrain crackers.

Second Afternoon snack (4 p.m.)

Handful of carrots and 4T hummus

Dinner (6 p.m.)

1 cup of homemade soup

1 cup of salad

Because this diet tightly controlled my blood sugar by restricting carbs in the latter half of the day, I could make it through the night without eating. I had to be militant about following it. Otherwise, I would be hungry in the evenings or worse, I would experience blood sugar lows any time I skipped a meal or snack.

I added free range eggs after a couple of weeks and started making omelets (soy milk, salt & pepper, fresh veggies and vegan cheese). Adding one or two ingredients a day, I figured out a reasonable diet plan for me and my son. He's a little luckier, and he can still eat my favorite snack food without symptoms: salt and vinegar potato chips. Alas, I cannot. Here is a typical day's food for me now; this may not work for you. For example, I can tolerate a small cup of half-caffeinated coffee, but caffeine can wreak havoc on a reactive hypoglycemic, so that's why it's so important to keep a food diary:

Sample Diet after one month

Breakfast (8 a.m.)

Small cup of ½ caffeinated, ½ decaffeinated coffee

1 slice of Ezekiel 4:9 raisin toast with butter

1 piece of fruit

Mid-morning snack (10 a.m.)

1 cup whole grain corn flakes

½ cup soy milk

Lunch (noon)

Stir fried vegetables, brown rice (1/4 cup) and beans

Afternoon snack (2 p.m.)

1 organic, live food bar

1 cup apple juice

Late afternoon snack (4 p.m.)

Handful of carrots and hummus

Dinner (6 p.m.)

1 cup chili

Handful of wholegrain, baked tortilla chips

Evening snack (8 p.m.)

1 cup frozen fruit

Bedtime (10 p.m.)

> *Evaporated cane juice* does not undergo the same refining process as regular sugar, and retains most of its nutrients and vitamins.

1 slice of Ezekiel 4:9 toast with peanut butter

I don't stick rigidly to the amount of food, although I do stick to the timing. If I miss a 2-hour meal I'll sometimes get grumpy and lightheaded. If I get hungry; I'll eat a few nuts or a small bowl of baked, whole-grain tortilla chips and salsa. I also take a multivitamin and a calcium supplement to make sure my symptoms aren't caused by a lack of calcium or fuddled by a vitamin deficiency.

I avoid any artificial sugars, but you may find them palatable. Personally, I prefer fructose, a type of sugar that does not raise my blood sugar (and therefore I do not experience a big drop). Fructose is typically 60% sweeter than regular sugar, so you can add less to recipes, like oatmeal cookies. That doesn't necessarily make it healthy—it's still a sugar, and not everyone will be able to tolerate it. I found both fructose and evaporated cane syrup (which I can also tolerate in small quantities) in my local health food store, and I have also been experimenting with xylitol, a natural sugar that also does not raise my blood sugar. I tried it in a stir fry recipe (replacing the brown sugar with it), and my whole family loved it. Xylitol can be found in your local health food store.

A List of Possible Foods

This list is comprised of products that should not cause you to have a hypoglycemic reaction. The foods in bold tend to be lower on the Glycemic Index (GI) and should be tolerated by everyone. Other foods listed are higher in the Glycemic Index; if you consume these be sure to balance your meal. For example, if you eat a ripe banana (high GI), balance it with a handful of nuts (high fat). Foods marked with an asterisk can be found in any health food store. Other foods on the list are foods that I introduced at a later time. You may differ in the foods that cause your blood sugar to elevate; keep a food diary to try and figure out your sensitivities, and don't eat multiple foods at once before you know for sure which ingredients you can tolerate well. For example, instead of having soup and salad for lunch, have the soup at noon and the salad at 2 p.m.. Splitting up foods like this will allow you to figure out what foods raise and crash your blood sugar, and which do not.

A note on serving sizes: I stuck to the serving sizes indicated on products during the first month. For example, Amy's soup has 2 servings in a can. One serving = one meal. If I was still hungry, I would eat a garden salad to fill me up (with one serving of salad dressing). I also began to buy almost exclusively organic products, because "regular" manufacturers have a nasty habit of sneaking in sugar and other unwanted substances into products. For example, I found sugar as an ingredient in Planter's dry roasted peanuts, sugar in Jif peanut butter, sugar and/or high fructose corn syrup in most supermarket wholewheat bread (including whole grain bread!), and the list goes on. Organic manufacturers seem to pride themselves in not using sugar or high fructose corn syrup and anyways, I got entirely tired of reading labels and looking up those alien sounding substances to figure out if I could eat them or not!

I included even innocuous sounding ingredients like baking powder. It was important for me to know *every ingredient* that was going into my body, because I thought it could be just that one small serving of an innocuous sounding ingredient that was setting me off. It turns out I was right: I cannot eat white bread products that contain evaporated cane juice. However, I can tolerate evaporated can juice in just about every other product. My best guess is that the carb load for white bread and can juice is just too high, and that my body needs to stay under a certain threshold.

Suggested Foods

Bold foods should be tolerated by all.

Asterisked * foods are available in health food stores.

All-Bran

Apple juice, no sugar added

Apples

Arrowhead Mills Graham Cracker Crust

Arrowhead Mills Kamut Flakes*

Baking powder

Balsamic vinegar

Bananas (ripe)

Bananas (slightly green)

Barley

Barley flakes

Bean Burgers (no bun)

Beans, dried and/or canned

Beets

Bob's Red Mill baking products*

Bran

Bread, Ezekiel 4:9

Bread, pumpernickel

Bread, sourdough

Breakfast cereal, organic, sweetened with evaporated cane juice or fruit juice*

Brown rice

Buckwheat groats*

Bulgur

Cappuccino (soy, decaf)

Carrots

Cheese, soy or rice products (no dairy)

Cherries

Chick peas

Chocolate chip cookies, vegan, sweetened with evaporated can

juice*

Citric acid

Coffee (half caf)

Coffee creamer, Silk (soy)

Corn tortillas

Cornstarch

Cream cheese, vegan, (try Tofutti brand)

Dill pickle

Dill relish (no sugar added)

Dressing, Amy's Gingerly Dressing

Dressing: Newman's Own Raspberry Vinaigrette

Dried Apricots

Edamame

Eggs (I only buy free range eggs)

Energy bars, raw food (i.e. Wild Bar)*

Flaxseed*

Flour, wholewheat

Fructose*

Fruit roll ups, 100% fruit, organic

Garden Salad

Garlic

Grapefruit

Grapefruit juice

Grapes

Green peas

Guacamole

Hamburger buns, Ezekiel 4:9

Herbs

Hot dogs, vegetarian, whole-wheat bun

Hummus

Indian curry

Jalapenos

Jelly, 100% fruit

Kashi 7-grain cereal puffs

Kavli crispy thin crackers*

Kiwi

Lentils

Mango

Miso soup

Morningstar Farms products (i.e. bean burgers, meatless crumbles)

Mustard

Nayonaise*

Nutritional yeast flakes

Nuts (plain or raw)

Oatmeal

Oils (I stick with olive oil mostly, sometimes canola and peanut for flavor)

Olives

Oranges

Peach

Peaches

Peanut butter

Pear

Pineapple juice

Plum

Plums

Quinoa

Quorn Chik'n Cutlets, unbreaded

Quorn nuggets, unbreaded,

Quorn products

Raw food bars*

Rolled oats

Roti (an Indian bread)

Ryvita dark rye crackers*

Salsa, organic

Salt

Sesame seeds

Soup, Amy's, all varieties

Sour Cream, vegan

Soy milk, sweetened with evaporated cane juice

Soy milk, unsweetened

Soy sauce

Soy yoghurt (sweetened with fructose or evaporated cane syrup)

Soybeans

Spaghetti & lasagna noodles, whole grain

Spaghetti Sauce, organic

Spices

Spread, vegan buttery

Strawberries

Sunflower seeds

Sushi (vegetable, 6 pieces)

Sweet potato fries

Sweet corn

Tabouli

Tahini

Tea, caffeinated

Tea, Herbal & decaffeinated

Tofu, any variety

Tofu, plain

Tofurkey sandwich slices

Tofutti ice cream

Tomato

Tomato juice and tomato sauce, organic

Tortilla, sprouted grain*

Vanilla extract

Vegenaise*

White potatoes in very small amounts (i.e. in soups)

White wine

Whole grain bagels and bread (without added sugar)

Wild rice

Xanitol*

Yam

Yeast

Food to Avoid

This list would not be complete without stating which foods should not be consumed. These are the most likely suspects that will raise your blood sugar faster than you can say High Fructose Corn Syrup. When I first starting purging my cupboards of anything that might be contributing to my reactive hypoglycemia, one of the first items to be purged from my kitchen was High Fructose Corn Syrup (HFCS). Americans consume more HFCS—an often genetically modified, cheap to produce product that has been linked to a host of disorders including diabetes—than real sugar. After reading about the complicated chemical process that is required to make HFCS, and how every dietician recommends that anyone with a blood sugar disorder should avoid HFCS, I set about purging my cupboards of the substance. Heinz Ketchup (I recently discovered that the organic version doesn't have HFCS). Pancake Syrup. Black Bean Soup. Some of our favorite products just had to go. We switched the pancake syrup for real berries, and the Black Bean Soup for Amy's organic soups. You can use HP sauce (a British steak sauce you can find in places like World Market) in place of ketchup.

I was dismayed to find that we had to completely change our diet. I had considered myself health conscious and used to purchase whole wheat and whole grain bread: you would rarely find a loaf of white in my cupboard. I knew white bread was a no-no for health, but whole grain bread sweetened with HFCS? Who would have thought? Here is a list of the top items I no longer consume.

Top Ten Foods to Avoid

1. *Supermarket bread products*: white bread, bagels, pizza, burger buns, or other "white" bread products. During the refining process, nearly all of the fiber and nutrients are lost.[51] Substitute whole grain products instead.

2. *White spaghetti noodles*: substitute whole grain products. Be careful to find "whole grain" and not wholewheat.

3. *Most breakfast cereals.* Apple Jacks was one of my son's favorite cereals until we read the label and discovered its #1 ingredient is sugar. Most cereals we find are completely unpalatable and cause a blood sugar reaction a couple of hours later. I can eat Arrowhead Mills Kamut Flakes, Oatmeal, All-Bran, and Kashi 7-grain cereal. Leo can eat a wider variety, but all come from the health food store and none have sugar or HFCS. He recently found a box of corn flakes sweetened with fruit juice that he loved.

4. *Anything that has "sugar" or "high fructose corn syrup" as an ingredient.* This sounds simple, but it really isn't. You'd be surprised at

where you find sugar: packaged meals, soups, canned beans, yoghurts, ice-cream, fruit cups, and baked goods. I stopped shopping at my local grocery store because of this problem. If I do go there, I stick to the produce aisle and the green/vegan section.

5. *Sodas and fruit juices.* The exception to this are tiny, one serving boxes of apple juice. I used to drink a wide variety of things, but now my list has diminished to a few products: water, coffee (one tiny cup in the morning), tea (mostly herbal) and apple juice on occasion. Anything else causes problems. I don't even drink diet drinks: they can have hidden caffeine, and I can't always trust myself to remember to check labels.

6. *Pastries, muffins, cakes, and other "treats":* There are a few treats I can have, including vegan chocolate chip cookies from my local health food stores. Why vegan? Chocolate chips in regular cookies are usually made with sugar: vegan cookies are usually made with homey, fructose, or evaporated cane sugar (which is as close to the plant as you can get). Those products I can tolerate in small amounts.

7. *Restaurant meals:* I avoid eating anything in a restaurant unless I am 100% certain that sugar is not one of the ingredients. This is such a problem that I rarely eat at restaurants anymore. There are exceptions: Indian food never causes me a problem (Indians tend not to add sugar to their meals), Sweet

Tomatoes/Soup Plantation (you can't beat a salad buffet), most items in Greek restaurants (except white pita) and vegetable fajitas at our local Mexican restaurant (I skip the tortillas and use corn chips instead). I can also eat tortilla chips and salsa in seemingly unlimited quantities. Not so good for me, but so delicious.

8. *White potatoes, including baked potatoes and fries*: except in small amounts, in a soup for example. I completely gave up trying to have these in my diet. They are just too high in sugars for me to be able to tolerate them: I substitute a small portion of sweet potato fries, and sometimes make sweet potato chili fries.

9. *High fat meats:* when I first tried to control my reactive hypoglycemia, I went on a strict vegan diet. I had read about the benefits of such a diet, and it worked wonders for me. I am now vegetarian. You can substitute low-calorie, nutrient dense products like Quorn, vegan burger crumbles, tofu, bean burgers, Tofurkey, and other meat analogues.

10.   *Potato chips and tortilla chips*. Leo can eat potato chips: I cannot. We can both eat tortilla chips, but that bad habit (full of carbs and not much else) may catch up to us someday. Instead, we substitute baked, whole grain tortilla chips (available at most grocery stores in the health food section).

Chapter 7: Internet Resources and Further Reading

Recommended books

You can purchase all of these books at my store at

http://www.reactivehypoglycemia.info/reactive-hypoglycemia-store/

The Reactive Hypoglycemia Cookbook. Stephanie Kenrose. ISBN 978-0-557-07047-3

The Reactive Hypoglycemic Cookbook has everything from slow cooker chili to fast French fries; there are plenty of family friendly meals that everyone can enjoy! With a whole section of slow cooker recipes, plus fun food, treats, and delectable entrees like spinach lasagna rolls and enchiladas, you won't feel like you're doing "without."

Baumel, S. *Dealing with Depression Naturally.* Lincolnwood, Illinois: Keats Publishing. 2000

Has a lot of useful information on reactive hypoglycemia (covered in Chapter 4), which can cause depression. Covers a staggering range of therapies. Full of information on natural antidepressant research, there are natural remedies abound, including correct nutrition bright light therapy and St. John's Wort. I recommend this book for anyone who wants to take an alternate route to allopathic medicine. If you are looking to treat your reactive hypoglycemia without drugs, this is the book to get.

Duyff, R. *American Dietetic Association complete food and nutrition guide.* Hoboken, NJ: Wiley & Sons. 2006.

This is the best nutrition book out there. If you are confused about what to eat, this book has it all. Although it doesn't *specifically* cover reactive hypoglycemia, it does offer a wealth of information on what types of food are good for you, what you should avoid, and what the Glycemic Index is all about.

Raine, A. (1993). *The psychopathology of crime: Criminal behavior as a clinical disorder.* San Diego, CA: Academic Press.

This fascinating book is worth a read, even though it only has a tiny amount of information on reactive hypoglycemia (including information on the link between reactive hypoglycemia and prison riots).

Internet Resources

Articles on everything Reactive Hypoglycemia, diet, causes, website reviews, reactive hypoglycemia store, and more.

http://www.reactivehypoglycemia.info

Basic info about Reactive Hypoglycemia from the Mayo clinic.

A good resource to direct friends and relatives to for a quick overview.

http://www.mayoclinic.com/health/reactive-hypoglycemia/AN00934

Basic info on Dumping Syndrome from the Mayo Clinic

http://www.mayoclinic.com/health/dumping-syndrome/DS00715/

Pathophysiology of the Digestive System.

Everything you ever wanted to know about what happens to the food you eat!!

http://arbl.cvmbs.colostate.edu/hbooks/pathphys/digestion/index.html

"Do You Have Undiagnosed Reactive Hypoglycemia?"

http://thyroid.about.com/b/2004/04/28/do-you-have-undiagnosed-hypoglycemia.htm

Overview of reactive hypoglycemia.

Article can be a bit confusing, because it interchanges the words "reactive hypoglycemia" and "hypoglycemia" but nonetheless has some good information.

http://emedicine.medscape.com/article/122122-overview

University of Dusseldorf website.

If you can get past the awkward language, this website has some **interesting facts**, including explaining the prediabetes-reactive hypoglycemic possible link.

http://www.uni-duesseldorf.de/MedFak/insulinoma/english%20homepage/mainpage/subpage/Epostpran_hypo.htm#top

Jean-Frédéric Brun's Website

This researcher specializes in exercise, fuel metabolism assessment in vivo, and hemorheology. You will find an excellent **academic paper** here about postrprandial reactive hypoglycemia and its causes.

http://jeanfrederic.brun.free.fr/postprandial%20hypo%20review%20diabetes%20metab.pdf

The article on **H-Pylori's effect on producing reactive hypoglycemia** can be found online.

http://www.springerlink.com/content/j231l47rx4n611j2/

Everything you ever wanted to know about the **Glycemic Index**.

http://www.glycemicindex.com/

Hypoglycemia Homepage Holland.

Full of **general information** on reactive hypoglycemia.

http://www.hypoglykemie.nl/

Personal Story on **Panic Disorder** and hypoglycemia.

http://www.hastingspress.co.uk/hypo/

Sample Menu for Reactive Hypoglycemia

http://www.dialadietitian.org/nutritionpage.asp?id=1391

Eating Guidelines for Reactive Hypoglycemia

http://www.dialadietitian.org/nutritionpage.asp?id=1280

Use of **Guar Gum** to Prevent Alcohol Induced Reactive Hypoglycemia

http://alcalc.oxfordjournals.org/cgi/content/abstract/16/3/135

Info on the "gin and tonic" effect on reactive hypoglycemia. Full article is available with a free subscription.

CBS News Story: **"Diabetes Sufferers: Beware of Caffeine"**
http://www.cbsnews.com/stories/2008/01/29/health/webmd/main37 63964.shtml

Armenian website with information on a **variety of different causes** for reactive hypoglycemia, including gastroectomy and alcohol-induced reactive hypoglycemia.

http://www.health.am/db/more/postprandial-hypoglycemia-reactive-hypoglycemia/

Nearly all of the articles and journals are available through your local library through interlibrary loan. Ask your local public library about it.

Appendix B: Complete Directory of Holistic Physicians Listed By State

I have researched literally hundreds of physicians listed by state and organized them for you in my book. By working with both your current doctor and a holistic doctor vet you could give yourself the edge you need to rapidly overcome your disease through a broad approach.

Alabama

Thomas Barrett, ND 119 Madison St. Alexander City, Alabama 35010
Phone: 256-414-4355 Email: jarvisclinic@bellsouth.net

David Fullwe, DO, FAAO, ABIHM Bay Minette, AL 251-937-7910

Linda Jarvis, NMD 1489 Slaughter Road Madison, Alabama 35758
Phone: 256-837-3448 Email: drtombarrett@charter.net
Web: www.drlindajarvis.com

Arizona

Karsten Alexandria, LAc ND 1420 E. Northern Ave. Phoenix, Arizona
85020 Phone: 602-938-8200 Email: doctorkarsten@yahoo.com
Web: www.doctorkarsten.com

Gladys Ceballos-Logan, NMD 1757 E. Baseline Road Bldg 9 Ste 135 Gilbert, Arizona 85233 Phone: 480-503-HEAL (4325) Email: heal@healability.com Web: www.healability.com

Jessica K. Anderson, NMD 7320 E. Deer Valley Rd Scottsdale, Arizona 85255 Phone: 480-513-2888 Email: dr.jessica.anderson@dermacare.com

Kristy L. Anderson, NMD 26705 S. 195th Street Queen Creek, Arizona 85242 Phone: 480-229-1348 Email: andersonaz02@yahoo.com

Jorge Cochran, NMD ND 310 N Wilmot Rd Suite 206 Tucson, Arizona 85711 Phone: 520-546-3233 Web: www.drcochran.meta-ehealth.com

Kyle Ann Cronin, ND 9200 E. Raintree Drive Ste 150 Scottsdale, Arizona 85260 Phone: 480-451-6161 Web: www.naturopathicgroup.com

Lila Flagler, NMD 6737 E. Camino Principal #C Tucson, Arizona 85715 Phone: 520-721-8821 Email: LilaFlagler@aol.com Web: www.DrFlagler.com

Julie Gorman, NMD LAc 3201 N. 3rd St. Phoenix, Arizona   85012 Phone: 602-265-1774 Email: info@aimcenteraz.com Web: www.AIMcenterAZ.com

Elizabeth K. Grady, NMD 130 West River Rd. Bldg A Tucson, Arizona 85704 Phone: 520-877-2668 Email: ekgnmd@earthlink.net Web: www.northsidenaturopathic.com

Louise D. Gutowski, NMD 7426 E. Stetson Dr. Suite 125 Scottsdale, Arizona   85251 Phone: 480-425-0800 Email: Lgutowski@aol.com Web: www.homeopathydoctor.ws

Danite Haller, ND 1250 E Baseline RD STe. 104 Tempe, Arizona   85283 Phone: 480-456-0402 Web: www.naturopathichealthassociates.com

Natalie Ham, ND 8010 E. McDowell Rd Suite 111 Scottsdale, Arizona Phone: 480-970-0000 Email: n.ham@scnm.edu

Clark H. Hansen, NMD 8070 East Morgan Trail Ste. 120 Scottsdale, Arizona   85258 Phone: 408-991-5092 Email: info@drhansen.com Web: www.DoctorHansen.com

Tikey Health, ND 13402 N. Scottsdale Rd. Bldg. B Ste 150 Scottsdale, Arizona 85254 Phone: 480-951-1248 Web: www.wellnessnmd.com

Judy A. Hiell, NMD 1 W. Wetmore Tucson, Arizona 85705 Phone: 520-887-4287 Email: drjudynmd@earthlink.net Web: www.drjudynmd.com

Janice Lynn Highfield, NMD 8010 E McDowell Rd Scottsdale, Arizona 85257 Phone: 480-970-0000 Email: j.highfield@scnm.edu Web: www.scnm.edu

Colleen Huber, NMD 1250 East Baseline Rd. Tempe, Arizona 85283 Phone: 480-839-2800 Email: office@naturopathyworks.com Web: www.naturopathyworks.com

Yu-Ree Hyun, NMD MA 9316 E. Raintree Dr. Ste. #140 Scottsdale, Arizona 85260 Phone: 480-614-2322 Email: yrhyun@gmail.com Web: www.sncaz.com

Hanna Ian, NMD MS 15436 West Statler Circle Surprise, Arizona 85374 Phone: 623-792-8889 Email: thenaturaldoctor@cox.net Web: www.thenaturopathicphysician.com

Suneil Jain, NMD 8390 E. Via de Ventura Suite F-111 Scotttsdale, Arizona 85258 Phone: 480-951-0111 Email: info@drsuneiljain.com Web: www.drsuneiljain.com

Suneil Jain, NMD 9977 N. 95th St. Suite 101 Scottsdale, Arizona 85258 Phone: 480-551-9000 Email: info@drsuneiljain.com

Andrew Kaufmann, ND PO Box 1651 San Carlos, Arizona 85550 Phone: 928-475-5924 Fax: 928-475-3118 Email: akaufmann@scatcom.net

Dana Keaton, LAc ND 906 W. McDowell Phoenix, Arizona 85007 Phone: 602-266-4670 Email: drkeaton@cox.net Web: www.centerfornaturalmedicine.com

Laura Kennedy, NMD MS 920 Black Drive Prescott, Arizona 86305 Phone: 928-445-4995 Email: lauraport@yahoo.com Web: www.myhealthwalk.com

Nita J. Keskitalo, ND 4035 W. Chandler Blvd. Chandler, Arizona 85226
Phone: 480-705-9611 Web: www.ChampionNH.com

Sarv Varta Kaur Khalsa, NMD 2480 W. Ray Rd. Suite 1 Chandler, Arizona
85224 Phone: 480-722-2811 Email: info@arizonanaturalmedicine.com
Web: www.aznaturalmedicine.com

Sandy Lutrin, ND RN 2912 East Sherran Lane Phoenix, Arizona 85016
Phone: 602-330-2278 Email: info@doctorlutrin.com
Web: www.doctorlutrin.com

Susy Macsay, NMD DDS 4333 N. Civic Center Plaza, Ste. 500 Scottsdale,
Arizona 85251 Phone: 480-231-4525 Email: dr.susy@yahoo.com
Web: www.WholisticAlivenessTraining.com

Lance J. Morris, ND 1601 N. Tucson Blvd. #37 Tucson, Arizona 85716
Phone: 520-322-8122 Email: wfmedicine@qwest.net
Web: www.drmorris.meta-ehealth.com

Joni Olehausen, ND 8010 East McDowell Road Scottsdale, Arizona
85257
Phone: 480-222-9834 Email: j.olehausen@scnm.edu
Web: www.scnm.edu

Andria Orlowski, ND 2655 West Guadalupe Mesa, Arizona 85202
Phone: 480-777-0445 Email: orlowskiNMD@msn.com
Web: www.innerlighthealth.com

Shahrzad Z. Orona, NMD 7517 S. McClintock Dr., Suite 201 Tempe,
Arizona 85283 Phone: 480-755-0060 Email: dr.orona@gmail.com
Web: www.drorona.com

Tara Peyman, NMD 5416 East Southern Avenue Ste 110 Mesa, Arizona
85206 Phone: 480-985-0000 Email: admin@DrTaraPeyman.com
Web: www.DrTaraPeyman.com

Tara Peyman, NMD 1250 E. Baseline Rd., Ste. 104 Tempe, Arizona
85283
Phone: (480) 456-0402 Email: admin@DrTaraPeyman.com
Web: www.DrTaraPeyman.com

Kenneth J. Proefrock, ND 9887 W. Bell Rd. Sun City, Arizona   85351
Phone: 623-977-0077 Web: www.novelRx.com

Jonathan Psenka, NMD 13832 N. 32nd Street #126 Phoenix, Arizona
85032 Phone: 602-493-2273 Email: 4wecare@gmail.com
Web: www.4wecare.com

Kristy Ratcliff, NMD Tempe, Arizona   85283 Phone: 480-244-6488
Email: drkris@privatehealthcarenow.com
Web: www.privatehealthcarenow.com

Stacy Riseborough, ND 1425 W. Elliot Rd Gilbert, Arizona   85233
Phone: 480-812-9000 Email: stacyrise@cox.net

Carrie Rittling, ND 5416 E. Southern Ave. Ste. 110 Mesa, Arizona   85202
Phone: 480-985-0000 Email: carrierittling@hotmail.com
Web: www.eastvalleynd.com

Herbert Schuck, ND 6767 N. 7th Street #220 Phoenix, Arizona   85014
Phone: 602-524-9768 Web: www.reachforhealing.com

Jason Sherbondy, NMD 876 N McQueen Rd Suite 108 Gilbert, Arizona
85233 Phone: 480-503-1977 Email: DrJason@HermosaMedical.com
Web: www.HermosaMedical.com

Margie Simmons-Stuber, NMD RN 4840 E Downing Circle Mesa, Arizona
85205 Phone: 480-396-3122 Email: DrMargSS@yahoo.com

Shaida Sina, ND 851 S. Main St. Suite E Cottonwood, Arizona   86326
Phone: 928-649-0269 Email: Info@gaiamedicine.com
Web: www.Gaiamedicine.com

Janice Skelton, NMD 13402 N Scottsdale Rd. Ste A-130 Scottsdale AZ,
Arizona   85254 Phone: 480-607-1277 Web: www.myriadwellness.com

Tam Spat, ND PhD 4700 S. McClintock Ste 105 Tempe, Arizona   85282
Phone: 480-222-2198 Web: www.naturehealing.com

Mary Ann Stalke, NMD ND 11989 N 93rd St Scottsdale, Arizona   85260
Phone: 480-703-5477 Email: dr.stalker@yahoo.com
Web: www.doctorsofnaturopathicmedicine.com

Stephanie Stark, ND 4646 E Ft Lowell Rd Suite 107 Tucson, Arizona 85712 Phone: 520-322-WELL (9355) Email: info@blueoakclinic.com Web: www.BlueOakClinic.com

Farra Swan, ND MA 2435 E Southern Suite 8 Tempe, Arizona 85282 Phone: 480-820-0911 Email: farraswan@aol.com

Tara Sae-In Swartz, NMD 16655 N. 90th Street Scottsdale, Arizona 5260 Phone: 480-991-5555 Web: www.naturopathicwellnesscenter.com

Katie Swedrock, ND 633 E. Ray Rd. Gilbert, Arizona 85296 Phone: 480-510-1747 Web: www.ndheal.com

David Dallas Thomason, NMD 906 W. McDowell Road Phoenix, Arizona 85007 Phone: 602-230-5350 Email: mynaturecare@gmail.com Web: www.zenmedicine.com

Jeannette Toghyani, ND 17007 E. Colony Dr. #102 Fountain Hills, Arizona 85268 Phone: 602-793-5828 Email: drtoghyani@treeoflifenaturopathic.com Web: www.treeoflifenaturopathic.com

Shana Turrell, ND 809 N. Humphreys Flaggstaff, Arizona 86001 Phone: 928-774-1770 Web: www.flagstaffnaturopathic.com

Michael Uzick, ND 2122 N. Craycroft Rd. Ste. 124 Tucson, Arizona 85712 Phone: 520-546-2321 Email: druzick@comcast.net Web: www.DoctorUzick.com

Teresa Vesco, ND 5533 E. Bell Rd. #116 Scottsdale, Arizona 85254 Phone: 602-996-8864 Web: www.anh.meta-ehealth.com

Sunshine Weeks, NMD 2666 S. Rural Rd Tempe, Arizona 85282 Phone: 480-921-9530 Web: www.solsanahealing.com

Laura Weeshoff, NMD 4960 S. Alma School Rd. #21 Chandler, Arizona 85248 Phone: 480-883-8160 Email: Leweeshoff@hotmail.com Web: www.azwellnessdoc.com

Wendy Wells, NMD 14301 N. 87th Street Scottsdale, Arizona   85260
Phone: 480-607-0299 Email: naaturdoc@yahoo.com
Web: www.drwendywells.com

Mercedes Williams, ND 13402 N. Scottsdale Road Scottsdale, Arizona
85254 Phone: 480-607-7999 Web: www.alternativesinhealth.com

Kimberly Wilson, NMD 2185 N Mosley Drive Chandler, Arizona   85225
Phone: 480-221-5296 Web: www.innovationsfps.com/wellness.html

Tracy Wooten, NMD 3714 E. Indian School Rd Phoenix, Arizona   85018
Phone: 602-840-4112 Email: tracy@palmvalleynd.com

Donese Worden, NMD MAPLC 6638 E. Baseline Rd. Mesa, Arizona
85206
Phone: 480-588-2233 Email: wordenmedicalspecialties@hotmail.com
Web: www.wordenmedicalspecialties.com

Valeria Wyckoff, NMD RD LLC 1257 W. Warner Road Suite B-4
Chandler, Arizona   85224 Phone: 480-857-2768 Email: drvaleria@att.net
Web: www.drvaleria.net

Alaska

Emily Kane, LAc ND 418 Harris Street #329 Juneau, Alaska   99801
Phone: 907-586-3655 Fax: 907-586-4326 Web: www.DrEmilyKane.com

Jennifer Lush, ND 915 W Northern Lights Anchorage, Alaska   99503
Phone: 907-770-6700 Fax: 907.770.6707 Email: drjlush@gmail.com
Web: www.avantemedical.com/practitioners/lush.html

L. Hope Wing, ND 3330 Eagle Street Anchorage, Alaska   99503
Phone: 907-561-2330 Fax: 907-561-1282 Email: rickhope82@yahoo.com

Adam Grove, ND 3330 Eagle Street Anchorage, Alaska   99516
Phone: 907-561-2330 Fax: 907-561-1282 Email: drgrove@ak.net

Jason Harmon, ND 915 W. Northern Lights Anchorage, Alaska   99503
Phone: 907-770-6700 Fax: 907-770-6707
Email: drharmonnd@yahoo.com

Patrick Huffman, ND 1020 East Rd Homer, Alaska   99603
Phone: 907-260-7725 Fax: 907-235-3691
Email: phuffmannd@hotmail.com

Kaycie Rosen, ND 915 W. Northern Lights Anchorage, Alaska   99507
Phone: 907-770-6700 Email: kaycierosen@hotmail.com

Toby Wheeler, ND PO Box 2289 Homer, Alaska   99603
Email: tobyw@xyz.net

Daniel Young, Lac ND 10928 Eagle River Rd Ste 254 Eagle River, Alaska
99577 Phone: 907-694-5522 Fax: 907-694-5524
Email: eagledoc@mtaonline.net

Conradine Zarndt, ND c/o 4341 TiKishla St. Anchorage, Alaska   99504
Phone: 503-780-4284 Email: czarndt@hotmail.com

Arkansas

Ann Arouh, ND 2800 S. University Little Rock, Arkansas   72204
Phone: 501-664-4886 Fax: 501-280-3255

Tara Hickman, NMD 345 St. Charles Ave Fayetteville, Arkansas   72703
Phone: 479-445-2220 Web: www.nwanaturalhealth.com

California

Heartfelt Medicine 2 1120 Via Miraleste Palm Springs, California   92262
Phone: 760-279-2134 Web: www.heartfeltmedicine.com

Willits Health 175 S. Humboldt St Willits, California 95490
Phone: 707-459-8500 Web: www.willitshealth.com

Koren Barrett, ND 1831 Orange Avenue Costa Mesa, California   92627
Phone: 949-642-3424 Email: drbarrett@inaturalmedicine.com
Web: www.inaturalmedicine.com

Arlan Cage, LAc ND MSOM 2204 Torrance Blvd. Torrance, California
90501 Phone: 310-803-8803 Email: info@southbaytotalhealth.com
Web: www.southbaytotalhealth.com

Christina Campbell, ND DC PO Box 6869 Tahoe City, California   96145
Phone: 530-583-0002 Email: doctorcampbell@sbcglobal.net
Web: www.tahoenaturalhealth.com

Trevor Cates, ND 34 E. Sola St. Santa Barbara, California   93101
Phone: 805-966-3003 Web: www.sbcnm.com

Dana Churchill, NMD 11704 Wilshire Blvd Los Angeles, California
90025
Phone: 310-230-5228 Email: drchurchill@heartfeltmedicine.com
Web: www.heartfeltmedicine.com

Dorothea Cist, ND 33533 Vista Colina Dana Point, California   92629
Phone: 949-429-7118 Web: www.thedorotheaclinic.com

Rita M. Conway, ND 1194 Pacific St. Ste 100 San Luis Obispo, California
93401 Phone: 805-781-9111 Web: www.doctorbagheri.com

Leigh-Anne Fraley, ND 501 Cedar Street Ste. B Santa Cruz, California
95060 Phone: 831-425-9900 Email: fraleynd@sbcglobal.net
Web: www.scienzen.com

Dennis Godby, ND MA 1507 21st St Suite 101 Sacramento, California
95814 Phone: 916-446-2591 Email: drgodby@diabetesnpc.com
Web: www.YourProgressiveHealthCare.com

Moses D. Goldberg, ND Santa Rosa, California   95403
Phone: 707-284-9200 Email: docmosesnd@yahoo.com
Web: www.docmoses.com

David Graves, ND 256 E. Hamilton Ave. Suite F Campbell, California
95128 Phone: 408-379-0133 Email: davidgravesnd@gmail.com
Web: www.familynd.com

Carl S. Hangee-Bauer, LAc ND 1615 20th St. San Francisco, California
94107 Phone: 415-643-6600 Email: Carl@sfnatmed.com
Web: www.sfnatmed.com

David Hogg, ND 1101 S. Winchester Blvd San Jose, California   95128
Phone: 408-297-6877 Email: drdavid@naturally4health.com
Web: www.naturally4health.com

Kasia Hopewell, ND 1601 El Camino Real Belmont, California   94002
Phone: 650-591-WELL (9355) Web: www.hopewellmedicine.com

Dorine Karlin, LAc ND 2104 Wilshire Blvd Santa Monica, California
90403
Phone: 949-375-1183 Email: dorinekarlin@gmail.com
Web: www.lotusew.com

Tara Levy, ND 2342 Almond Avenue Concord, California   94520
Phone: 925-602-0582 Web: www.taranaturalmedicine.com

John Lynch, ND 7222 Owensmouth Ave. #100 Canoga Park, California
91303 Phone: 818-222-2037 Email: GetWell979@yahoo.com
Web: www.johnlynchnd.com

Luc M Maes, ND DHANP DC 9 E Mission Street Santa Barbara,
California   93101 Phone: 805-563-8660 Email: doctor@maescenter.com
Web: www.maescenter.com

Samia McCully, ND 841 El Camino Real Menlo Park, California   94025
Phone: 650-233-7327 Web: www.wellnessarchitecture.com

Manqun Merry, Li LAc 370 San Bruno Ave West # F San Bruno,
California   94066 Phone: 650-588-8335 Email: merry@merryclinic.com
Web: www.merryclinic.com

Melissa N. Metcalfe, ND 890 Hampshire Rd. Suite B Westlake Village,
California   91361 Phone: 805-374-7363
Email: dr.melissa@naturalsolutions.com Web: www.naturalsolutions.com

John K. Monagle, NMD 1004 Magnolia Avenue Larkspur, California
94939 Phone: 415-366-7450 Email: drjohn@marinnatural.com
Web: www.marinnatural.com

Jaspreet Mundeir, ND 140 Gregory Lane Pleasant Hill, California   94523
Phone: 925-812-4990 Email: Drjmundeir@gmail.com
Web: www.suratnaturopathic.com

Nicole M. Ortiz, ND Palm Desert, California Phone: 971-404-9735
Email: dr.ortiz@livewellclinic.org Web: www.livewellclinic.org

Lisa Ow, ND 680 E. Romie Lane Salinas, California   93901
Phone: 831-771-5500 Email: reception@SalinasNaturalHealth.com
Web: www.SalinasNaturalHealth.com

Karen Peters, ND Albany, California   94706 Phone: 510-926-9987
Email: drkpeters@gmail.com Web: www.eastbaynaturopathic.com

Andrea Purcell, NMD 1770 Orange Avenue Costa Mesa, California
92627
Phone: 949-722-6797 Web: www.portaltohealing.com

Caroline Radosz, ND 1456 San Pablo Ave Berkeley, California   94702
Phone: 510-773-6058 Email: info@BerkeleyND.com
Web: www.BerkeleyND.com

Elspeth Gwynne Seddig, ND 4255 18th Street Suite 202 San Francisco,
California   94114 Phone: 415-921-2123 Web: www.naturopathic-sf.com

Keegan Sheridan, ND 2001 S Barrington Avenue Los Angeles, California
90025 Phone: 310-270-7918 Email: k.sheridan@evolvinghealth.com
Web: www.evolvinghealth.com

Aimée Gould Shunney, ND 501 Cedar Street Santa Cruz, California   95060
Phone: 831-335-3500 Email: ags@drshunney.com
Web: www.drshunney.com

Mark Stengler, ND 8950 Villa La Jolla Drive La Jolla, California   90237
Phone: 858-450-7120 Email: mark@lajollawholehealth.com
Web: www.lajollawholehealth.com

Kristin Stiles Green, ND 2811 Wilshire Blvd Santa Monica, California
90403 Phone: 310-453-2335 Web: www.lifespanmedicine.com

Suzanne Tang, LAc ND 3140 Bear St. #200 Costa Mesa, California
92626
Phone: 714-429-0838 Email: drtang@empoweredhealthcenter.com
Web: www.empoweredhealthcenter.com

Nirvana Tehranian, ND 1391 Warner Ave. Tustin, California   92780
Phone: 949-836-6991 Email: DrNirvana@tustinwellness.com
Web: www.drnirvana.com

Tou Vue, ND MS 15575 La Honda Sur Morgan Hill, California   95037
Phone: 408-779-7000 Email: DrVyasND@yahoo.com
Web: www.DrVyasND.tripod.com

Rajesh Vyas, LCEH ND. 15575 La Honda Sur Morgan Hill, California
95037
Phone: 408-779-7000 Web: www.DrVyasND.tripod.com

Abida Zohal Wali, ND 3257 Camino De Los Coches Carlsbad, California
 92009 Email: dr.wali@opintegrativecenter.com
Web: www.opintegrativecenter.com

Suzann Wang, ND 616 University Avenue Palo Alto, California   94301
Phone: 650-327-2053 Email: drswang@naturalhealthcalifornia.com
Web: www.naturalhealthcalifornia.com

Suzann Wang, ND 3030 Bridgeway Sausalito, California   94965
Phone: 415-331-1823 Email: drswang@naturalhealthcalifornia.com
Web: www.naturalhealthcalifornia.com

Louisa L. Williams, ND 2144 Fourth Street San Rafael, California   94901
Phone: 415-460-1968 Email: louisawilliams@mac.com
Web: www.radicalmedicine.com

Darcy Yent, LAc ND MSOM 2602 1st Avenue, Suite 209 San Diego,
California   92103 Phone: 619-501-5654 Email: drdarcymarie@aol.com
Web: www.drdarcy.meta-ehealth.com

Minna Yoon, N.D. L.Ac. 919 Irving St. Suite 104 San Francisco, California
 94122 Phone: 415-722-6680 Email: minnayoon@hotmail.com
Web: www.baynaturalmedicine.com

Colorado

Clinix Healing Center 7030 S. Yosemite Suite 210 Centennial, Colorado
80112 Phone: 303-996-3249 Web: www.clinixusa.com

Ruth Adele, ND 1625 W Uintah St. Suite I Colorado Springs, Colorado
80904 Phone: 719-636-0098 Email: RuthAdele@aol.com

Celeste Aurorean, ND 318 East Main Street Cortez, Colorado   81321
Phone: 970-739-8367 Email: drceleste@animas.net

Hilary Back, LAc ND 20 N. 4th Street Carbondale, Colorado   81623
Phone: 970-963-6500 Email: clientresources@drhilaryback.com
Web: www.drhilaryback.com

Jason E. Barker, ND 1103 Oak Park Drive Fort Collins, Colorado   80525
Phone: 970-237-1062 Web: www.DrJasonBarker.com

Faith A Christensen, ND RN 1010 W Colorado Ave Ste D Colorado
Springs, Colorado   80904 Phone: 719-651-4383
Email: drfaithnd@hotmail.com Web: www.springsnaturalmedicine.com

Jenny Demeaux, RNC ND 3441 Tennyson St Denver, Colorado   80212
Phone: 303-433-5006 Email: theHighlandsND@msn.com
Web: www.HighlandsHealthandHealing.com

Tara Skye Goldin, ND 2825 Marine St. #203 Boulder, Colorado   80303
Phone: 303-443-2206 Email: taraskye@juno.com
Web: www.taraskyegoldin.com

Brenna Hatami, ND 1441 York Street Ste 303 Denver, Colorado   80206
Phone: 303-320-1174 Web: www.doctorbrenna.com

Mark Kelley, LAc ND 209 East Swallow Road Fort Collins, Colorado
80525
Phone: 970-223-7425 Web: www.kindermedicine.com

Eliza Klearman, ND 407 Broadway Eagle, Colorado   81631
Phone: 970-328-5678 Web: www.drklearman.com

Janine Malcolm, LAc ND 2760 29th St. Suite 2E Boulder, Colorado
80301
Phone: 303-541-9600 Email: naturedocj@hotmail.com
Web: www.naturalresourceshealthcare.com

Rhonda Marcus, ND 3113 S. Taft Hill Road Fort Collins, Colorado   80526
Phone: 970-672-7771 Email: Rhondamarcusnd@comcast.net

Lynn McGuire, ND 2885 Aurora Ave, Suite 29 Boulder, Colorado   80303
Phone: 303-447-1339 Email: info@bouldernatural.com
Web: www.bouldernatural.com

Kelly J. Parcell, ND 5330 Manhattan Circle Boulder, Colorado   80303
Phone: 303-884-7557 Email: kelly@naturemedclinic.com
Web: www.naturemedclinic.com

Nancy A. Rao, LAc ND 1295 Yellow Pine Ave Boulder, Colorado   80304
Phone: 303-545-2021 Email: nancyraond@comcast.net
Web: www.drprattnd.com

Debra Rouse, ND 24230 Matterhorn Drive PO Box 587 Indian Hills,
Colorado   80454 Phone: 303-697-6662 Email: bealiveandwell@aol.com
Web: www.optimumwellness.com

James Ellis Rouse, ND PO Box 587 Indian Hills, Colorado   80454
Phone: 303-697-6662 Email: optimumwellness1@aol.com
Web: www.optimumwellness.com

Jacob Schor, ND 1181 S Parker Rd Denver, Colorado   80231
Phone: 303-337-4884 Email: jacob@denvernaturopathic.com
Web: www.denvernaturopathic.com

Abigail Seaver, ND 123 S. Laura St. Ridgway, Colorado   81432
Phone: 970-626-3188 Email: abigailseaver@yahoo.com
Web: www.drabigailseaver.com

Mary Shackelton, ND 2975 Valmont Rd. Suite 100 Boulder, Colorado
80301 Phone: 303-449-3777 Email: mary@allnaturaldoc.com
Web: www.allnaturaldoc.com

Jody K. Shevins, ND DHANP 5377 Manhattan Circle Boulder, Colorado
80303 Phone: 303-494-3713 Email: shevins@qwest.net

Kathleen Young, ND 2121 Academy Circle S Suite 100 Colorado Springs,
Colorado   80909 Phone: 719-238-6816 Email: drkyoung@comcast.net

Connecticut

West Hartford Naturopathic Medicine LLC 301 North Main Street West
Hartford, Connecticut   06117 Phone: 860-232-9662
Email: Draieta@aol.com Web: www.draieta.com

Ather Ali, ND MPH 252 Seymour Avenue Derby, Connecticut 06418
Phone: 203-732-1370 Email: shelli.larovera@yalegriffinprc.org
Web: www.imc-griffin.org

Debra Anastasio, ND 286 Maple Avenue Cheshire, Connecticut 06410
Phone: 203-271-1311 Web: www.nenaturopathic.com

Cynthia L Anderson, ND RN MS 3519 post Rd Southport, Connecticut
06890 Phone: 203-254-2633 Web: www.sabitaholisticcenter.com

Ann Aresco, ND 355 New Britain Rd. Kensington, Connecticut 06037
Phone: 860-829-0707 Email: draresco@comcast.net
Web: www.kensingtonnaturopathic.com

Michael Armentano, ND 296 Sound Beach Ave Greenwich, Connecticut
06870 Phone: 203-637-8464 Email: drarmentano@att.net
Web: www.drarmentano.com

Alice P. Bell, ND MS 415 Howe Ave. Suite 307 Shelton, Connecticut
06484 Phone: 203-922-0029 Web: www.naturohealthcenter.com

Joshua K Berry, ND 31 Hawleyville Rd Hawleyville, Connecticut 06440
Phone: 203-426-2306 Email: drjoshnd@gmail.com
Web: www.hawleyvillenaturopathic.com

Stephanie Bethune, ND 107 Wilcox Road Ste 103 Stonington, Connecticut
06378 Email: drstephaniebethune@gmail.com
Web: http://www.snhc.com

Mistie Charles, ND 213 Danbury Road Wilton, Connecticut 06897
Phone: 203-834-7500 Web: www.dadamo.com/wordpress

Peter J. D'Adamo, ND 213 Danbury Road Wilton, Connecticut 06897
Phone: 203-834-7500 Web: www.dadamo.com/wordpress

Lisa Gengo, ND 8 Knight St. Norwalk, Connecticut 06851
Phone: 914-419-7585 Email: ljgnd@optonline.net

Debra A. Gibson, ND 158 Danbury Road Ridgefield, Connecticut 06877
Phone: 203-431-4443 Email: dgnd2006@sbcglobal.net

Karl M. Goldkamp, LAc MSOM 81 Halls Road Old Lyme, Connecticut
06371 Phone: 860-434-3100 Email: drgoldkamp@sbcglobal.net
Web: www.center4naturalmedicine.com

Pearlyn Goodman-Herrick, ND PC 1465 Post Rd. E. Westport, Connecticut 06880 Phone: 203-256-9091 Email: goodmanherrick@aol.com

Carolyn U. Graham, ND RN 415 Howe Avenue Suite 307 Shelton, Connecticut 06484 Phone: 203-922-0029
Web: www.naturohealthcenter.com

Gary Gruber, ND PC 68 Old Stamford Road New Canaan, Connecticut 06840 Phone: 203-966-6360 Email: gsgruber@optonline.net
Web: www.sciencemeetsnature.com

Lynnette M. Guida, LAc ND 670 Newfield Street Middletown, Connecticut 06457 Phone: 860-347-8800 Email: docguida@yahoo.com
Web: www.avalonhealingcenter.net

Sharon Hunter, ND 777 Farmington Avenue West Hartford, Connecticut 06119 Phone: 860-232-0000 Email: shunter@center4health.com
Web: www.connecticutcenterforhealth.com

Jennifer L Johnson, ND Bridgeport, Connecticut 06604
Phone: 203-576-4425 Web: www.drjenjohnson.com

Guru Sandesh Singh Khalsa, ND 60 Lafayette St. Bridgeport, Connecticut 06604 Phone: 203-576-4110 Email: gkhalsa@bridgeport.edu
Web: www.bridgeport.edu

Christine Kontomerkos, ND MS 88 Noble Avenue Suite 104D Milford, Connecticut 06460 Phone: 203-874-4333
Email: NaturalHealth_Doc@yahoo.com Web: www.letnatureheal.com

Jenn Krebs, ND 26 Trumbull Street New Haven, Connecticut 06511
Phone: 203-776-1212 Web: www.drjennkrebs.com

Amanda M Levitt, ND 3011 Whitney Ave. Hamden, Connecticut 06518
Phone: 203-288-8283 Email: amandameisel@yahoo.com
Web: www.wholehealthct.com

Joshua Levitt, ND 3011 Whitney Ave Hamden, Connecticut 06518
Phone: 203-288-8283 Email: drjlevitt@yahoo.com
Web: www.wholehealthct.com

Margot Longenecker, ND 850 North Main Street Extension Wallingford, Connecticut Web: www.connecticutcenter4health.com

Cassandra Mannhardt, ND RN 25 Court Street New Britain, Connecticut 06051 Phone: 860-229-1490 Web: www.avonwellnesscenter.net

Alison L Monette, ND 243A Kennedy Drive Putnam, Connecticut 06260 Phone: 860-963-2250 Email: avenawellness@gmail.com Web: www.avenawellness.com

Artemis D. Morris, LAc ND MS 867 Whalley Avenue New Haven, Connecticut 06515 Phone: 203-387-1540 Email: revivewellness@aol.com Web: www.revivewellnesscenter.com

Artemis D. Morris, LAc ND MS 87 Cherry Street Milford, Connecticut 06460 Phone: 203-783-9802 Email: revivewellness@aol.com Web: www.revivewellnesscenter.com

Stacey Munro, ND 96 Poquonock Avenue Windsor, Connecticut 06095 Phone: 860-688-2275 Email: info@natureshelpermedical.com Web: www.NaturesHelperMedical.com

Ginger Nash-Wolfe, ND LLC 21 Anderson Street New Haven, Connecticut 06511 Phone: 203-777-7911 Email: gingernash@gmail.com Web: www.gingernash.com

Natural Solutions for Health Robin Ritterman, LAc ND 494 Glenbrook Rd. Ste 3 Stamford, Connecticut 06906 Phone: 404-755-2291 Email: msamm@doctor.com

Amy B. Rothenberg, ND DHANP 115 Elm St Enfield, Connecticut 06082 Phone: 860-763-1225 Web: www.nesh.com

Andy L. Rubman, ND 900 Main St. South Southbury, Connecticut 06488 Phone: 203-262-6755 Web: www.naturopath.org

James S. Sensenig, ND 2558 Whitney Avenue Hamden, Connecticut 06518 Phone: 203-230-2200 Fax: Fax: 203-230-1454 Web: www.naturalhealthct.com

Christina Shannon, ND 148 East Avenue Norwalk, Connecticut 06851 Phone: 203-523-5600 Email: DrShannon@TLCMedicine.com Web: www.TLCMedicine.com

Victoria Shikhman, ND 144 Morgan Street Ste 1 Stamford, Connecticut 06905 Phone: 203-323-0500 Email: victoriashik@gmail.com Web: www.WhiteOakMedical.com

Lisa Singley, ND MS 88 Noble Avenue Suite 104 Milford, Connecticut 06460 Phone: 203-874-4333 Email: info@nhawc.com Web: www.nhawc.com

Veronica Waks, ND 992 High Ridge Rd. 3rd Floor Stamford, Connecticut 06905 Email: drvwaks@yahoo.com Web: www.drwaks.com

Keith Zeitlin, ND 850 North Main St. Ext Wallingford, Connecticut 06492
Phone: 203-284-1119 Web: www.5elementsnhc.com

Tina M. Zigo, ND 188 Main St. Suite E Monroe, Connecticut 06468 Phone: 203-268-1336 Email: c.healing@sbcglobal.net Web: www.ctrnaturalhealing.com

Victoria Zupa, ND 397 Post Rd. Darien, Connecticut 06820 Phone: 203-656-4300 Email: Zupaorders@cs.com Web: www.victoriazupa.com

Florida

Michelle E. Clark, ND 537 Fore Drive Bradenton, Florida 34208 Phone: 941-747-0627 Email: info@askdoctorclark.com Web: www.AskDoctorClark.com

Katherine Clements, ND LMT 3131 S. Tamiami Trail Sarasota, Florida 34239 Phone: 941-951-6820 Email: DrClementsND@aol.com Web: www.auroratherapeudics.com

Steven DAntonio, ND 635 Primera Blvd. Lake Mary, Florida 32746 Phone: 407-333-1059 Email: DoctorStevenND@aol.com Web: www.cflhealthandwellness.com

Jessica Lipham, LAc ND 2700 South Tamiami Trail Sarasota, Florida 34239 Phone: 941-780-7738 Email: drjessicalipham@yahoo.com Web: www.geocities.com/drjessicalipham

Kimberly Nguyen, LAc ND MBA 6328 Gunn Hwy Suite C Tampa, Florida 33625 Phone: 813-774-4392 Email: bvclinic@yahoo.com Web: www.bvclinic.com

Rob Streisfeld, NMD 7785 Travelers Tree Dr Boca Raton, Florida 33433 Phone: 866-650-3200 Email: docrob@phdpros.com Web: www.phdunlimited.com

Rob Streisfeld, NMD 7785 Travelers Tree Dr Boca Raton, Florida 33433 Phone: 866-650-3200 Email: docrob@phdpros.com Web: www.phdunlimited.com

Katie Swedrock, ND Miami Beach, Florida Phone: 786-999-9695 Email: swedrock@ndheal.com Web: www.ndheal.com

Michael Visconti, LAc ND MSOM 235 Citrus Tower Blvd. Clermont, Florida 34711 Phone: 352-241-7581 Email: info@docvisconti.com Web: www.docvisconti.com

Georgia

Martha Allen, LAc ND MSOM The Leather's Building Athens, Georgia 30601 Phone: 706-424-4219 Email: marthamea@msn.com

Bradley Bongiovanni, ND 3502 Old Milton Pkwy Alpharetta, Georgia 30005 Phone: 678-879-4242 Email: drb@wmsoa.com Web: www.wmsoa.com

Winston B. Cardwell, LAc ND MSOM 5755 North Point Parkway Alpharetta, Georgia 30022 Phone: 678-218-4230 Email: wcardwell@spherios.com Web: www.rethinkyourhealth.com

John B. Davis, ND 3756 Lavista Rd. Suite 104 Tucker, Georgia 30084 Phone: 404-325-7734 Email: docjbd@aol.com

Wyler Hecht, LAc ND 1612 Mars Hill Rd. Ste C Watkinsville, Georgia 30677 Phone: 706-769-8300 Email: wyler@nc.rr.com Web: www.LeilasApothecary.com

Maureen Flora Melendrez, ND 4340 Georgetown Square Atlanta, Georgia 30338 Phone: 770-451-1966 Email: drmelendrez@aol.com Web: www.mydrmelendrez.com

Alane M. Palmer, ND CNC 45 West Crossville Road, Suite 501 Roswell, Georgia   30022 Phone: 678-372-2913 Email: alanepnd@aol.com Web: www.nutritionallyyours.net

Hawaii

Nicole J. Baylac, ND 17-502 Ipuaiwaha Street Keaau, Hawaii   96749 Phone: 808-982-8202 Email: retreat@mindyourbody.info Web: www.mindyourbody.info

Carrie Brennan, ND 4-1558 Kuhio Hwy Kapaa, Hawaii   96746 Phone: 808-652-7581 Email: carriejbrennan@hotmail.com Web: www.drcarriebrennan.com

Margaret Dexter, N.D. 79-7393 Mamalahoa Hwy Suite #9 Kainaliu, Hawaii 96750 Phone: 808-322-0055 Email: mdexternd@gmail.com

Catherine Downey, ND POB 968 Kilauea, Hawaii   96754 Phone: 808-828-6153 Email: catherine@laolahealth.com Web: www.LaOlaHealth.com

Jenna L Dye, ND 81-6587 Mamalohoa Hwy Bldg A Kealakekua, Hawaii 96750 Phone: 808-323-3370 Email: dr.jdye@gmail.com

Veronica Ford, ND MS 408 Uluniu Street Kailua, Hawaii   96734 Phone: 808-261-6244 Email: VMFordND@hawaii.rr.com Web: www.BodyWizeHawaii.com

Mary Lynn Garner, ND 47-4628 Waipio Road Honokaa, Hawaii   96727 Phone: 808-775-1505 Email: hawaiind@BigIsland.net Web: www.naturopathicretreatcenter.com

Julie Claire Holmes, ND 2846 Omaopio Road Kula, Hawaii   96790 Phone: 808-878-3267 Email: jholmesnd@hawaii.rr.com Web: www.DrJulieHolmes.com

Lori Kimata, ND 1188 Bishop Street Honolulu, Hawaii   96813 Phone: 808-783-0361 Web: www.sacredhealingarts.info

Laurie A. Steelsmith, LAc ND 438 Hobron Lane Ste. V-6 Honolulu, Hawaii   96815 Phone: 808-943-0330 Web: www.drsteelsmith.com

Sarah Bronwyn Strong, ND 152 Puueo St Hilo, Hawaii   96720
Phone: 808-933-HEAL (4325) Email: doc@drsarahstrong.com
Web: www.drsarahstrong.com

Karen Tan, ND MAcOM LAc 320 Ward AVe Suite 105 Honolulu, Hawaii
  96814 Phone: 808-591-8778 Web: www.drkarentan.com

Michael L. Traub, ND 75-5759 Kuakini Hwy # 202 Kailua-Kona, Hawaii
96740 Phone: 808-329-2114 Web: www.balancerestored.com

Jason Uchida, ND 615 Piikoi Street Honolulu, Hawaii   96814
Phone: 808-589-1955 Web: www.drjasonuchida.com

Idaho

Gabrielle Duebendorfer, ND 101 N 4th Ave Suite 106 Sandpoint, Idaho
83864 Phone: 208-265-2213

Joan Haynes, ND 4219 W. Emerald Boise, Idaho   83706
Phone: 208-338-0405 Web: www.boisenaturalhealth.com

Pamela Langenderfer, NMD LAc 520 Coeur D'Alene Ave. Coeur D'Alene,
Idaho   83814 Phone: 208-664-1644 Email: drpamelasue@verizon.net
Web: www.naturalmedicinecda.com

Sara Rodgers, ND MS 4219 W Emerald St. Boise, Idaho   83706
Phone: 208-338-0405 Web: www.boisenaturalhealth.com

Mario Roxas, ND 301 1/2 First Avenue Suite #208 Sandpoint, Idaho
83864 Phone: 208-946-0984 Email: info@drroxas.com
Web: www.drroxas.com

Mario Roxas, ND 25820 Highway 2 West Dover, Idaho   83825
Phone: 800-228-1966 Email: info@drroxas.com Web: www.drroxas.com

Todd A. Schlapfer, ND 520 Coeur D'Alene Avene Coeur D'Alene, Idaho
83814 Phone: 208-664-1644 Email: tasnd@aol.com

Mika Tsongas, ND LAc MSOM 120 E Lake St, Suite 205 Sandpoint,
Idaho   83864 Phone: (208) 255-1951
Email: mtsongas@greenmtmed.com Web: www.greenmtmed.com

Chante Wiegand, ND 65 S Main St Suite 6 Driggs, Idaho   83422
Phone: 208-354-9579 Web: www.pangeanaturalhealth.com

Illinois

Chad D. Aschtgen, ND at Midwestern Regional Medical Center
Zion, Illinois   60099 Phone: 847-731-4156
Email: chad.aschtgen@ctca-hope.com Web: www.cancercenter.com

Shauna M. Birdsall, ND Midwestern Regional Medical Center Zion,
Illinois 60099 Phone: 847-872-6444 Email: shaunabirdsall@ctca-
hope.com Web: www.cancercenter.com

Tim C. Birdsall, ND 2520 Elisha Ave Zion, Illinois   60099
Phone: 847-872-6067 Email: tim.birdsall@ctca-hope.com
Web: www.cancercenter.com

Helen Davakos, ND DC 4727 Willow Springs Rd. Unit 3S La Grange,
Illinois   60525 Phone: 708-482-1099 Email: davakos@integrativefha.com
Web: www.integrativefha.com

Stephanie Draus, ND 2519 N California Avenue Chicago, Illinois   60647
Phone: 773-486-3797 Email: stellariachicago@yahoo.com
Web: www.stellarianaturalhealth.com

Julie E. Martin, ND 2520 Elisha Ave Zion, Illinois   60085
Phone: 847-731-4126 Web: www.cancercenter.com

Jin Park, LAc ND MSOM 3111 Dundee Rd Northbrook, Illinois   60062
Phone: 847-562-0840 Web: www.integratemed.com

Andrew R. Peters, ND DC 1012 W. Fairchild Street Danville, Illinois
61832
Phone: 217-443-4372 Email: info@illinoisnaturalhealth.com
Web: www.illinoisnaturalhealth.com

Preety A Shah, ND 3200 S Harlem Ave Riverside & Saint Charles, Illinois
  60546 Phone: 630-456-0640 Email: preetyshah@gmail.com
Web: www.ndsource.com

Preety A Shah, ND 1409 E Palatine Rd. Arlington Heights, Illinois   60004
Phone: 630-456-0640 Web: www.ndsource.com

Lidia Wiersum, ND 2520 Elisha Ave Zion, Illinois   60099
Phone: 847-746-7178 Email: lidia.wiersum@ctca-hope.com

Indiana

Deborah Lightstone, ND 1033 Sagamore Parkway West West Lafayette,
Indiana   47906 Phone: 765-463-3000 Email: dlightstone@gmail.com
Web: www.docdeb.net

Emily Moore, LAc ND 200 High Park Ave Goshen, Indiana   46526
Phone: 574-535-2888 Web: www.cancermidwest.com

Marcia Prenguber, ND MS 200 High Park Ave. Goshen, Indiana   46526
Phone: 574-535-2961 Web: www.cancermidwest.com

Iowa Jacqueline Stoken, DO, ABIHM West Des Moines
Phone: 515 327 0046

Kansas

Amber Belt, ND 901 Kentucky Lawrence, Kansas   66044
Phone: 785-218-0606 Email: amberbeltnd@yahoo.com
Web: www.amberbeltnd.com

Deena Beneda-Khosh, ND 4824 Quail Crest Place Lawrence, Kansas
66049 Phone: 785-749-2255

Michael Brown, ND 11240 Strangline Road Lenexa, Kansas   66215
Phone: 913-498-0005 Fax: 877 303-0762
Email: physicianschoiceks@msn.com Web: www.physicianschoiceks.biz

Chad Krier, ND DC 3100 N. Hillside Wichita, Kansas   67219
Phone: 316-682-3100 Email: ckrier@brightspot.org
Web: www.brightspot.org

William Ryan Shelton, ND 11791 W 112th Street Overland Park, Kansas
66210 Phone: 913-961-6308 Email: drshelton@wholebodyhealth.com
Web: www.wholebodyhealth.com

Kentucky

Carol Perkins, ND 509 Southland Drive Lexington, Kentucky   40503
Phone: 859-277-5255 Email: drbunny01@hotmail.com
Web: www.natural-choices.info

Chase Ann Roth, LAc ND 161 Chenoweth Lane Louisville, Kentucky
40207
Phone: 502-410-8363 Email: chaseroth@insightbb.com

Louisiana

Erin Holston Singh, ND Shreveport, Louisiana Phone: 318-675-3676

Maine

Sarah T. Ackerly, ND 53 Main Street Topsham, Maine   04086
Phone: 207-798-3993 Web: www.northernsunfamilyhealthcare.com

Julie Barter, ND 69 Elm Street Suite 104 Camden, Maine   04843
Phone: 207-230-113 Web: www.nfmedicine.com

Laura T. Bridgman, ND 179 Main St. Waterville, Maine   04901
Phone: 207-859-8711

Julianne M. Forbes, ND MBA 120 North Bridgton Rd North Bridgton,
Maine   04057 Phone: 207-647-9423 Email: jmforbesnd@gmail.com
Web: www.mainenaturopath.net

Devra M. Krassner, ND 153 US Route 1 Scarborough, Maine   04074
Phone: 207-883-5517 Email: dkrassner@maine.rr.com
Web: www.mainewholehealth.com

Christopher J. Maloney, ND 4 Drew St. Augusta, Maine   04330
Phone: 207-623-1681 Email: docleroymaloney@hotmail.com
Web: www.maloneymedical.com

Fredric Shotz, ND 222 Auburn Street Portland, Maine   04103
Phone: 207-828-4299 Email: drshotz@mainewellness.com

Priscilla D. Skerry, ND 260 Western Avenue South Portland, Maine 04106 Phone: 207-772-5227

Maryland

Seeds Center for Whole Health 3600 Roland Avenue Baltimore, Maryland 21211 Phone: 410-235-1776 Web: www.seedswellness.com

Nazirahk K.K. Amen, ND 7120 Carroll Ave. Takoma Park, Maryland 20912
Phone: 301-891-2488 Web: www.doctoramen.com

Rachel M. Anderson, ND 115 Ridgely Ave Annapolis, Maryland 21401
Phone: 410-268-2025 Email: drrachelmanderson@gmail.com
Web: www.AnnapolisNaturalHealth.com

Rachel M. Anderson, ND 115 Ridgely Ave Annapolis, Maryland 21401
Phone: 410-268-2025 Email: drrachelmanderson@gmail.com
Web: www.AnnapolisNauralHealth.com

Stephanie Becker, ND 2014K Renard Ct. Annapolis, Maryland 21401
Phone: 202-457-8282 Email: drsjbecker@aol.com
Web: www.naturalmedicine-wccm.com

Stephanie Becker, ND 900 19th Street NW Washington District of Columbia, Maryland 20006 Phone: 202-457-8282
Email: drsjbecker@aol.com Web: www.naturalmedicine-wccm.com

Veronica E. Hayduk, ND 912 Thayer Ave. Silver Spring, Maryland 20910
Phone: 301-395-9118 Email: veronica@drveronicahayduk.com

Veronica E. Hayduk, ND 620 Hungerford Dr. Suite 15 Rockville, Maryland 20850 Phone: 301-395-9118
Email: veronica@drveronicahayduk.com
Web: www.secondnaturehealth.com

Daemon Jones, ND 8630 Fenton St Silver Spring, Maryland 20910
Phone: 301-608-0670 Email: info@healthydaes.org
Web: www.healthydaes.org

Giselle Lai, LAc ND 252 E Sixth Street Frederick, Maryland 21701
Phone: 301-620-1557 Web: www.healingpowerofnature.com

Kevin Passero, ND 203 Ridgely Ave Annapolis, Maryland 21401
Phone: 443-433-5540 Web: www.greenhealingnow.com

Steven Sinclair, LAc ND 252 East 6th St Frederick, Maryland 21701
Phone: 301-620-1557 Web: www.healingpowerofnature.com

Emily Telfair, ND LMT 4711 Harford Road Baltimore, Maryland 21214
Phone: 410-254-2786 Email: dremilytelfair@gmail.com
Web: www.greatsoulwellness.com

Massachusetts

Anna Abele, ND 26 Market Street Northampton, Massachusetts 01060
Phone: 413-587-0122 Email: Anna@DrAbele.com
Web: www.DrAbele.com

Lisa Anne Arnold, ND 177 Cranberry Hwy Route 6A Orleans,
Massachusetts 02653 Phone: 508-255-9141
Web: www.DrLisaArnold.com

Theolinda Barry, ND MA 800 Providence Rd. Rte. 122 Whitinsville,
Massachusetts 01588 Phone: 508-234-5655
Email: drtbarry@verizon.net

Shiva Barton, LAc ND 10 Converse Place Winchester, Massachusetts
01890 Phone: 781-721-4585 Email: ShivaBartonND@verizon.net
Web: www.winchesternaturalhealth.com

Janet K. Beaty, ND MA LMT PO Box 661 Harvard, Massachusetts
01451
Phone: 978-456-7789 Email: janet@janetbeaty.com
Web: www.janetbeaty.com

Geffin Falken, ND 1073 Hancock St. Ste.103 Quincy, Massachusetts
02169 Phone: 617-689-3392 Email: gfalken@gmail.com
Web: www.drgeffinfalken.com

Rebecca Lawrence, ND 261 Waquoit Hwy Waquoit, Massachusetts 02536
Phone: 508-548-7373 Web: www.lawrencenatural.com

James Lemkin, ND 7 Cole Rd Haydenville, Massachusetts   01039
Phone: 413-268-3500 Email: jim@walkingattheedge.com

Oceana Rames, ND PO Box 4934 Vineyard Haven, Massachusetts   02568
Phone: 508-696-3992 Web: www.droceana.com

Peter Swanz, NMD 46 Pearl Street Cambridge, Massachusetts   02139
Phone: 617-388-5126 Email: drswanz@gmail.com
Web: www.vitalforcenaturopathy.com

Peter Swanz, NMD 320 Rindge Avenue Cambridge, Massachusetts   02140
Email: drswanz@gmail.com

Amanda Tracy, ND 790 Turnpike St North Andover, Massachusetts
01845 Phone: 978-327-5960 Email:drtracy@advancedhealthonline.com
Web: www.advancedhealthonline.com

Michigan

AnnAlisa Behling, ND in the Preventive Medicine Clinic Flint, Michigan
48502 Phone: 810-233-5300 Email: annalisand@yahoo.com
Web: www.naturespathmedical.com

Rami El-Hussieny, ND LMT 3448 East Lake Lansing Rd East Lansing,
Michigan   48823 Phone: 517-944-0116
Web: www.michiganholistics.com

Kim Palka, ND 2513 Louanna St. Ste #102 Midland, Michigan   48640
Phone: 989-633-0025 Web: www.wellspringnaturopathic.com

Julie TwoMoon, NMD LAc MSOM 44670 Ann Arbor Road Ste 110
Plymouth, Michigan   48170 Phone: 734-414-7669
Email: info@breathingwaters.net Web: www.breathingwaters.net

Jean Wagner, ND 425 Main St. Ste 201 Rochester, Michigan   48307
Phone: 248-881-6220 Web: www.JeanWagnerND.com

Minnesota

Lee Aberle, ND Sartell, Minnesota   56377 Phone: 320-253-4112
Email: naturallee@mac.com Web: www.NatFamMed.com

Rebecca Alderson, ND 3800 East 26th Street Minneapolis, Minnesota 55406 Phone: 612-226-6207 Email: heartfullhealing@gmail.com Web: www.midwestherbsandhealing.com

Rebecca Alderson, ND 2919 Pentagon Dr. St Anthony, Minnesota 55418 Phone: 612-781-3006 Web: www.midwestherbsandhealing.com

Kristin Becker, ND 775 Edmund Avenue St Paul, Minnesota 55104 Phone: 651-340-4145 Email: The_Natural_Path@yahoo.com Web: www.minnesotanaturalhealth.com

Helen C. Healy, ND 905 Jefferson Ave St. Paul, Minnesota 55102 Phone: 651-222-4111 Email: wellspringclinic@msn.com Web: www.helenhealynd.com

Rachel Roberts Oppitz, ND 17261 State Hwy 34 Park Rapids, Minnesota 56470 Phone: 218-237-2312 Email: dr.oppitz@itascaintegrative.com Web: www.itascaintegrative.com

Diaa Osman, ND MPH 2960 Winnetka Avenue North Crystal, Minnesota 55427 Phone: 763-546-3736 Email: drosman@backtolifehealth.com Web: www.backtolifehealth.com

Robin Thomson, ND 4801 Hwy 61 Suite 203 White Bear Lake, Minnesota 55110 Phone: 651-653-0170 Email: DrThomson@natfamilymed.com Web: www.natfamilymed.com

Mississippi

Willie C. Bell, ND 1331 Rockdale Dr. Jackson, Mississippi 39213 Phone: 601-906-4742 Email: williecbell64@yahoo.com

Missouri

Matthew Cowan, ND 2024 Cherry Hill Drive Ste. 101 Columbia, Missouri 65203 Phone: 573-447-1225 Email: drmatthewcowan@yahoo.com

Jody Krukowski, NMD 1810 Summit St Kansas City, Missouri 64108 Phone: 602-320-2990 Email: treatemnat@aol.com

Jamila Owens-Todd, ND 5705 Ramsey Drive St. Louis, Missouri   63136
Phone: 314-677-4041

Montana

Northwest Neuro-Cranial Medicine 266 Bear Canyon Rd Bozeman, Montana
59715 Phone: 425-330-6352

NBI Testing and Consulting Corp 1087 Stoneridge Drive Bozeman, Montana
59718 Phone: 800-NBI-1416 Web: www.nbitesting.com

Laura Barbosa, ND 1004 South Ave. Missoula, Montana   59802
Phone: 406-880-2454 Web: www.missoulanaturalcare.com

Margaret R. Beeson, ND LM 720 North 30th Street Billings, Montana
59101 Phone: 406-259-5096 Email: ync@180com.net
Web: www.yncnaturally.com

Marissa Cavalier, ND 1805 Bancroft St. Missoula, Montana   59801
Phone: 406-721-1632 Web: www.vitalhomeopathic.com

Paloma Defuentes, ND 9202 River Road Bozeman, Montana   59718
Phone: 406-599-9337 Email: doctorpalomand@yahoo.com
Web: www.mtnaturopathicclinic.com

Michael Lang, ND 9202 River Road Bozeman, Montana   59718
Phone: 406-586-1100 Email: michaellangnd@yahoo.com
Web: www.NaturesWisdom.info

John Neustadt, ND 1087 Stoneridge Drive Bozeman, Montana   59718
Phone: 406-582-0034 Email: drneustadt@montanaim.com
Web: www.montanaim.com

Deborah Oleynik, ND 910 7th Street South Great Falls, Montana   59405
Phone: 406-771-7114 Email: tnhc2003@yahoo.com

Lynn Troy, ND 305 First Ave. W Columbia Falls, Montana   59912
Phone: 406-892-2102 Web: www.lynntroynd.com

Christine C. White, ND 521 S. 2nd St. West Missoula, Montana   59801
Phone: 406-542-2147 Web: www.blackbearnaturopaths.com

Nebraska Randall Bradley, DHANP ND 7447 Farnam St Omaha, Nebraska   68114 Phone: 402-391-6714
Web: www.HeartlandNaturopathic.com

Nevada

Kemberly Bacon, ND 754 Mays Blvd #2 Incline Village, Nevada   89450
Phone: 775-832-2171 Email: drkemby@naturavitanv.com
Web: www.naturavitanv.com

Christopher Delellis, ND P.O. Box 4711 Incline Village, Nevada   89450
Phone: 775-832-2171 Email: drchris@naturavitanv.com
Web: www.naturavitanv.com

Jessica Edge, ND 3400 Kauai Court Suite 100 Reno, Nevada   89509
Phone: 775-827-6888 Email: jedgend@aol.com Web: www.rahcc.com

Tara Finley, LAc ND MSOM 6490 S. McCarran Blvd. Reno, Nevada 89509
Phone: 775-337-1334 Email: DrTaraFinley@yahoo.com
Web: www.thefinleycenter.com

Nichole Gardner, ND MS 3012 S. Durango Dr. Ste. 1 Las Vegas, Nevada 89117 Phone: 702-366-0640 Email: drgardner.nd@gmail.com

New York

Benjamin Asher, MD New York, NY 212-223 4225

Ohio

Yaser Abdelhamid, ND LAc 730 SOM Center Road #190 Mayfield Village OH 44143 , Ohio Phone: 440-995-0303
Email: info@MyWellnessEvolution.com
Web: www.MyWellnessEvolution.com

Jennifer Ball, ND 5115 Olentangy River Rd Columbus, Ohio   43235
Phone: 614-442-2336 Web: www.everythingismedicine.com

Shelley Bluett, ND 1680 Akron Peninsula Rd Akron, Ohio   44313
Phone: 330-928-6685 Email: drshelley@snwcenter.com
Web: www.snwcenter.com

Tamara Macdonald, LAc ND 1814-B Pearl Road Brunswick, Ohio   44212
Phone: 330-460-5155 Email:drtamara@northcoastnaturalhealth.com
Web: www.northcoastnaturalhealth.com

Nicholas Parasson, ND 1680 Akron Peninsula Road Akron, Ohio   44313
Phone: 330-928-6685 Email: drnick@snwcenter.com
Web: www.snwcenter.com

Erin Holston Singh, ND 2460 Fairmount Blvd. Suite 219 Cleveland
Heights, Ohio   44106 Phone: 216-707-9137
Email: docerin@optionsnaturopathic.com
Web: www.optionsnaturopathic.com

Lori Starn, ND P.O. Box 259 Pataskala, Ohio   43062 Phone: 740-964-
6920 Web: www.naturopathicpathways.com

Tamara E. Strickland, ND 5115 Olentangy River Rd. Columbus, Ohio
43235 Phone: 614-442-2336 Web: www.EverythingIsMedicine.com

Oklahoma

Katherine Anderson, ND 10109 E. 79th St. Tulsa, Oklahoma   74133
Phone: 908-286-5170 Email: katherine.anderson@ctca-hope.com

Markian Babij, ND 10109 E 79th Street Tulsa, Oklahoma   74133
Phone: 918-286-5775 Email: markian.babij@ctca-hope.com

Katrina Ariel Bogdon, ND 10109 E. 79th Street Tulsa, Oklahoma   74133
Phone: 918-286-5754 Email: katrina.bogdon@ctca-hope.com
Web: www.cancercenter.com

Letitia Cain, ND 10109 E 79th St Tulsa, Oklahoma   74133
Phone: 918-286-5170 Web: www.cancercenter.com

Daniel Lander, ND 10109 East 79th street Tulsa, Oklahoma   74133
Phone: 918-286-5173 Email: daniel.lander@ctca-hope.com

Andrea M. Lee, ND Midwest City, Oklahoma   73110 Phone: 480-363-
4501
Email: andrealeend@gmail.com

Michael D. Leu, ND RPh 407 W. A St Jenks, Oklahoma 74037
Phone: 918-298-9300 Email: leumike@msn.com Web: www.drleu.com

Oregon

Thomas Abshier, ND 1414 NE 109th Ave. Portland, Oregon 97220
Phone: 503-255-9500 Email: naturedox@qwest.net
Web: www.naturedox.com

Susan S. Allen, ND 2601 NE Glisan Street Portland, Oregon 97232
Phone: 503-232-1948 Email: drsusanallen@qwest.net
Web: www.triangolofamilyclinic.net

Rebecca Asmar, ND 838 SW First Avenue Suite 330 Beaverton, Oregon
97204 Phone: 503-274-9360 Web: www.bambuclinic.com

Amy Bader, ND 3808 N. Williams Suite F Portland, Oregon 97227
Phone: 1-800-738-7303 Email: amybadernd@comcast.net
Web: www.benourished.org

Steven Bailey, ND 1540 SE Clinton Street Portland, Oregon 97202
Phone: 503-224-8083 Email: bnatural@spiritone.com
Web: www.nwnclinic.com

Carrie Baldwin-Sayre, ND 1330 SE 39th Ave Portland, Oregon 97214
Phone: 503-232-1100 Email: drbaldwin-sayre@cnm-inc.com
Web: www.cnm-inc.com

Pauline Baumann, ND 1168 Butler Creek Road Ashland, Oregon 97520
Phone: 503-709-2188 Email: seroya@charter.net

Audrey Bergsma, ND 2220 SW 1st Ave. Portland, Oregon 97201
Phone: 503-552-1551 Email: abergsma@ncnm.edu

Rita M. Bettenburg, ND 10360 NE Wasco St Portland, Oregon 97220
Phone: 503-252-8125

Adrienne Borg, ND 74 East 18th Ave. Suite 12 Eugene, Oregon 97401
Phone: 541-686-3330 Email: aplusr@earthlink.net

David A Bove, LAc ND 1161 Lincoln Street Eugene, Oregon   97401
Phone: 541-683-2126 Email: docb@drbove.info Web: www.drbove.info

Elizabeth Busetto, ND LLC 711 NE Dekum St Portland, Oregon   97211
Phone: 503-789-7953 Email: drbusetto@gmail.com
Web: www.drbusetto.com

Petra Caruso, ND 4926 SE Woodstock Blvd. Portland, Oregon   97206
Phone: 503-771-0615 Email: drpetracaruso@comcast.net
Web: www.woodstockclinic.com

Loch Stephen Chandler, LAc ND MSOM 1st Floor North Tower Portland,
Oregon   97213 Phone: 503-215-3219
Email: loch.chandler@providence.org
Web: www.providence.org/integrativemedicine

Anya Chang, ND 8555 SW Tualatin Road Tualatin, Oregon   97062
Phone: 503-691-0901 Email: dranyachang@truehealthmedicine.com
Web: www.truehealthmedicine.com

Julie Anne Chinnock, ND MPH 1132 SW 13th Ave Portland, Oregon
97205 Phone: 503-535-3859 Email: juliec@outsidein.org

Jeffery J Clark, ND PO Box 23911 Tigard, Oregon   97224
Phone: 503-449-0476 Email: drjeffclark@TrueHealthMedicine.com
Web: www.TrueHealthMedicine.com

Joseph J. Coletto, N.D. L.Ac. P.C. 10525 SE Cherry Blossom Drive
Portland, Oregon   97216 Phone: 503-253-3443 x211
Email: joecoletto@comcast.net

Nicole Daddona, ND 1820 SW Vermont Street Portland, Oregon   97219
Phone: 503-307-3337 Email: nicole@salusnaturalmedicine.com
Web: www.salusnaturalmedicine.com

Joshua David, ND 8933 N. Lombard St Portland, Oregon   97203
Phone: 503-286-4400 Email: drdavidpdx@gmail.com
Web: www.stjohnshealthcenter.com

Bruce Dickson, ND DHANP 119 NE 3rd St McMinnville, Oregon   97128
Phone: 503-434-6515 Email: info@keytohealthclinic.com
Web: www.keytohealthclinic.com

Meredith Distante, ND 1608 SE Ankeny St. Portland, Oregon   97214
Phone: 503-313-0509 Email: dr.merrie@blossomnaturalhealth.com

Rob Dramov, ND 9735 SW Shady Lane #104 Tigard, Oregon   97223
Phone: 503-639-6454 Email: drrob@dramovmedical.com
Web: www.dramovmedical.com

Gary Carl Dreger, LAc ND 710 John Adams St. Oregon City, Oregon
97045 Phone: 503-722-7776 Email: drgary@qwest.net
Web: www.naturalhw.com

Shaun Vincent Dyler, LAc ND MSOM 14088 SW Odino Ct. Tigard,
Oregon   97224 Phone: 503-579-9493 Email: s.dyler@att.net
Web: drdyler.com

Dawson A. Farr, ND 504 ne jessup st Portland, Oregon   97211
Phone: 503-363-0524 Web: www.groundswellhealthcare.com

Cinda Flynn, ND 1220 NW Kings Blvd Corvallis, Oregon   97330
Phone: 541-753-5152 Email: cflynnnd@msn.com

Lindsay Fontenot, ND 125 NE Killingsworth St #101 Portland, Oregon
97211 Phone: 503-223-3741 Web: www.bloomnaturalhealthcare.com

Karen M. Frangos, ND 049 SW Porter Portland, Oregon   97209
Phone: 503-552-1814 Email: dr.frangos@naturopathicbodyworks.net
Web: www.naturopathicbodyworks.net

Arcoma Gonzalez Lambert, ND 1911 Mt View Ln Forest Grove, Oregon
97116 Phone: 503-357-2826 Email: drarcoma@blossominghealth.com
Web: www.blossominghealth.com

Mary Grabowska, LAc ND LM 2304 E Burnside St #104 Portland,
Oregon   97214 Phone: 503-236-6006 Email: mgrabowska@ncnm.edu
Web: www.naturopathic.org

David A. Greenspan, ND 6655 SW Hampton St. Ste 110 Tigard, Oregon
97223 Phone: 503-684-1875 Email: info@greenspangoodhealth.com
Web: www.greenspangoodhealth.com

Laurie Grisez, ND 497 SW Century Drive Bend, Oregon 97702
Phone: 541-389-6935 Web: www.bluestarclinic.com

Chikako Nishiwaki Harper, ND LMT 4085 SW 109th Ave #200
Beaverton, Oregon 97005 Phone: 503-477-0472
Email: info@DrChikakoHarper.com Web: www.DrChikakoHarper.com

Margaret Havlik, ND 22808 SW Forest Creek Dr #102 Sherwood,
Oregon 97140 Phone: 503-625-0320 Email: mhavlik.nd@gmail.com

Dianna Lynn Henson, ND 12125 NE Penny Lane Carlton, Oregon 97111
Phone: 503-864-4797 Email: www.doctordianna.com
Web: www.DoctorDianna.com

Dana Herms, ND 2604 SE 33rd Place Portland, Oregon 97202
Phone: 503-313-5930 Email: danaherms@yahoo.com

Kimberly Hindman, LAc ND 1820 SW Vermont Suite C Portland, Oregon
97219 Phone: 503-784-1027 Web: www.healingdragon.net

Geoff Houghton, ND 153 Clear Creek Dr. Suite 101 Ashland, Oregon
97520 Phone: 541-482-8484 Email: HoughtonND@aol.com

Tori S. Hudson, ND 2067 NW Lovejoy Portland, Oregon 97209
Phone: 503-222-2322 Email: womanstime@aol.com
Web: www.awomanstime.com

Michelle K. Jackson, ND PC 334 NE Irving Ave. Suite 103 Bend, Oregon
97701 Phone: 541-385-0775 Email: michelle@drjacksonnd.com

Amy Beth Johnson, ND 4729 SE 36th AVE Portland, Oregon 97202
Phone: 503-772-5316 Email: amynaturedoc@gmail.com

Tina Kaczor, ND 247 W. 10th Avenue Eugene, Oregon 97401
Phone: 541-338-9494 Email: info@clinicofnaturalmed.com
Web: www.clinicofnaturalmed.com

Stephanie Kaplan, ND 4031 SE Hawthorne Blvd Portland, Oregon 97214
Phone: 503-975-2617 Email: drkaplan@earthlink.net

Azure Dee Karli, ND 715 NW Hill St. Bend, Oregon 97701
Phone: 541-389-9750 Email: info@bendnaturopath.com
Web: www.bendnaturopath.com

Jorge Kaufmann, LAc ND MSOM 838 SW 1st Ave Portland, Oregon 97204
Phone: 503-274-9360 Email: www.bambuclinic.com

Heather Krebsbach, LAc ND 2348 NW Lovejoy St. Portland, Oregon 7210
Phone: 503-224-7224 Email: hkrebsbach@gmail.com

Roman Krupa, ND 4900 SE Division Portland, Oregon 97206
Phone: 503-445-9771 Email: drkrupa@urbanwellnesspdx.com
Web: www.urbanwellnesspdx.com

Angela Lambert, LAc ND 6434 N. Kerby Avenue Portland, Oregon 97217
Phone: 503-703-5019 Web: www.ahealingpath.org

Raina Lasse, ND 833 SW 11th Suite 214 Portland, Oregon 97205
Phone: 503-224-2525 Email: drlasse@redleafclinic.com
Web: www.redleafclinic.com

Alison McAllister, ND 4444 SW Corbett Ave Portland, Oregon 97239
Phone: 503-224-2590 Web: doctormcallister@gmail.com

Meredith McClanen, ND 6501 SE King Road Milwaukie, Oregon 97222
Phone: 5032564895 Web: drmimi@hotmail.com

Kristen McElveen, ND 2220 SW 1st Ave Portland, Oregon 97206
Phone: 503-552-1551 Email: drkristen@baremedicine.com
Web: www.baremedicine.com

Lissa McNiel, ND 3654 C South Pacific Highway Medford, Oregon 97501
Phone: 541-535-9200 Web: www.arboranms.com

Anthony Murczek, LAc ND MSOM 3449 N.E. 25th Ave. Portland, Oregon 97212 Phone: 503-528-1065
Email: tony@mountainspringhealth.com
Web: www.mountainspringhealth.com

Sheila M. Myers, ND 4390 NE Emerson Bend, Oregon 97701
Phone: 541-385-6249 Web: www.sagehealthcenter.com

Judy Neall, ND 1221 SE Madison Street Portland, Oregon   97214
Phone: 503-520-8859 Web: www.naturalchoicesclinic.com

Bonnie Lisette Nedrow, ND LM 815 Oak Street Ashland, Oregon   97520
Phone: 541-488-2233 Email: drbonnie@bonniend.com
Web: www.bonniend.com

Sara Ohgushi, ND 2304 E. Burnside Suite 101 Portland, Oregon   97214
Phone: 503-236-6006 Web: www.sarasfamilycare.com

Virginia Oram, ND 400 E 2nd Ave. Suite 105 Eugene, Oregon   97401
Phone: 541-343-2384 Web: www.droram.com

Mihaela Pepel, ND MD 15880 SW Quarry Road Lake Oswego, Oregon
97035 Phone: 503-232-3302 Email: drPepel@msn.com
Web: www.DrPepelFamilyPractice.com

Shawn Marie Peters, ND 2329 Pacific Avenue Forest Grove, Oregon
97116 Phone: 503-357-1706 Email: dr_shawn@fghealthandfitness.com
Web: www.fghealthandfitness.com

Heidi Peterson, ND MS 4444 SW Corbett Ave Portland, Oregon   97239
Phone: 503-224-2590 Web: www.doctorheidi.com

Noel S. Peterson, ND 560 First St. Suite 204 Lake Oswego, Oregon   97034
Phone: 503-636-2734 Web: www.myctm.org

Kristen Plunkett, ND 1200 NE 7th St Grants Pass, Oregon   97526
Phone: 541-476-2916 Email: dr.plunkett@yahoo.com

Kelley R. Reis, ND 172 SE 6th Ave Hillsboro, Oregon   97123
Phone: 503-693-0904 Email: drkelley_nd@yahoo.com
Web: www.hillsboronaturalmedicine.com

Lee Samatowic, ND 8600 SW Salish Lane, Suite One Wilsonville, Oregon
97070 Phone: 503-682-3811 Email: thewellnesspro@gmail.com
Web: www.thewellnesspro.com

Renee Schwartz, ND 11930 SW Greenburg Road Tigard, Oregon   97223
Phone: 503-639-1712 Email: RENEESND@EARTHLINK.NET
Web: www.tigardholistic.com

Janice Seibert, ND 2187 SW Main St #103 Portland, Oregon   97205
Email: drjanseibert@yahoo.com
Web: www.seiberthealthandwellness.com

Janice Seibert, ND 327 SE 3th Ave Hillsboro, Oregon Phone: 503-477-9340
Email: drjanseibert@yahoo.com Web: www.hormonerejuvenation.com

Angela Senders, ND 838 SW 1st Ave Portland, Oregon   97204
Phone: 503-274-9360 Email: drsenders@bambuclinic.com
Web: www.bambuclinic.com

Juliette Soihl, ND 4838 NE Sandy Blvd. Suite 200 Portland, Oregon 97213
Phone: 503-287-1510 Web: www.centerforvibranthealth.com

Mitchell Bebel Stargrove, LAc ND 4720 SW Watson Ave. Beaverton, Oregon   97005 Phone: 503-526-0397
Web: www.wellspringofhealth.com

Ananda Stiegler, ND 295 West Broadway Eugene, Oregon   97405
Phone: 541-653-8881 Email: drananda@balanceinhealth.com
Web: www.balanceinhealth.com

Michelle M Sturm, LAc ND MSOM 1211 N. Webster Street Portland, Oregon   97217 Phone: 503-351-5426
Email: drmichelle@thehousesofhealing.com
Web: www.thehousesofhealing.com

Augusta Gusty Swift, ND 6018 SE Stark St. Suite 103 Portland, Oregon 97215 Phone: 503-239-6698 Email: drswift@vitalhealthpdx.com
Web: www.vitalhealthpdx.com

Wendy D. Vannoy, ND 2067 NW Lovejoy St. Portland, Oregon   97209
Phone: 503-222-2322 Email: womanstime@aol.com

Jacqueline Villalobos, ND 85 N. 12th Cornelius, Oregon   97113
Phone: 503-359-5564 Email: jvillalobos@vgmhc.org
Web: www.virginiagarcia.org

Serron Wilkie, ND 4804 SE Lincoln St Portland, Oregon 97215
Phone: 503-956-9396 Email: drserronwilkie@me.com

Kevin C. Wilson, ND 328 West Main Street Suite C Hillsboro, Oregon
97123 Phone: 503-648-0484 Email: kcwnd@teleport.com
Web: www.kevinwilsonnd.com

Sara Wood, ND 4085 SW 109th Ave. Ste. 200 Beaverton, Oregon 97005
Phone: 503-643-1024 Email: sara.wood@comcast.net
Web: www.beavertonnaturopathicmedicine.com

Carol Ann Zamarra, ND LMT 8113 SE 13th Ave Portland, Oregon
97202
Phone: 503-232-5653 Email: drzamarra@ghcenter.com
Web: www.ghcenter.com

Texas

Chriselda Beltran, ND San Antonio, Texas 78299 Phone: 602-750-6106
Email: naturaldoc@earthlink.net

Erica Campbell, NMD LMT 5411 Morningside Dr. Houston, Texas
77005
Phone: 713-529-Well Email:DrCampbell@VillageHerbsandWellness.com
Web: www.VillageHerbsandWellness.com

Stacy Dunn, LAc ND MSOM Dallas, Texas 75219 Phone: 214-520-8108
Email: info@wellnaturalhealth.com Web: www.wellnaturalhealth.com

Jeanne Galloway, ND 801 W. 34th Street Austin, Texas 78705
Phone: 512-695-2342 Email: GallowayHealth@msn.com
Web: www.GallowayNaturalHealth.com

Dr Jonci Jensen, ND 2003 S. Lamar Suite 12 Austin, Texas 78704
Phone: 512-586-6834 Email: drjonci@gmail.com Web: www.drjonci.com

Roger Fletcher Kies, ND 8930 Four Winds Drive Suite 206 San Antonio,
Texas 78239 Phone: 210-767-1767 Email: rfknd@yahoo.com

Melanie Landers, ND 4910 Burnet Road Austin, Texas 78756
Phone: 512-320-0200 Email: drmlanders@msn.com
Web: www.austinnaturalhealth.com

Carol McCalment, ND 19002 FM 1488 Magnolia, Texas   77355
Phone: 713-303-0808 Email: naturaldocsoftx@aol.com

Carol A McCalment, ND 19002 FM1488 Magnolia, Texas   77355
Phone: 281 259-5850 or 713 303-0 Email: naturaldocsoftx@aol.com

Melanie Meyer, ND MS 21332 Provincial Blvd. Katy, Texas   77450
Phone: 281-650-0405 Email: drmeyer@wellnatured.com
Web: www.wellnatured.com

Amy Neuzil, ND 5524 Bee Caves Rd Austin, Texas   78746
Phone: 512-306-0373 Email: dramy@excelonhealth.com
Web: www.excelonhealth.com

Rhonda Jane Steinke, ND 108 West 38 St. Austin, Texas   78705
Phone: 830-265-4921 or 512-669-1 Web: www.healthtn.org

Kimberly Wilson, NMD MBA 6545 Preston Road Suite 200 Plano, Texas
75024 Phone: 972-608-0100 Email: contact@innovationswellness.com
Web: www.innovationswellness.com

Utah

Matthew Burnett, LAc ND 242 South 400 East Suite A Salt Lake City,
Utah   84111 Web: www.utahnaturalmedicine.com

Rachel Burnett, LAc ND 242 South 400 East Suite A Salt Lake City, Utah
84111 Phone: 801-363-UTAH (8824)
Web: www.utahnaturalmedicine.com

Joe J. Holcomb, ND 1870 N. Main St. #206 Cedar City, Utah   84720
Phone: 435-586-4854 Web: www.cedarnaturalhealth.com

Thaddeus E. Jacobs, LAc ND MSOM Salt Lake City / Park City, Utah
Phone: 435-647-9500 Email: drtjacobs@summitintegrative.com
Web: www.summitintegrative.com

Ulrich G. Knorr, ND 2188 S. Highland Dr. #207 Salt Lake City, Utah
84106
Phone: 801-474-3684 Email: uliknorr@mac.com
Web: www.eastsidenaturalhealth.com

Leslie J. Peterson, ND 150 S. 600 E. Ste 6B Salt Lake City, Utah   84102
Phone: 801-746-3555 Web: www.fullcirclecare.com

Katherine Ruggeri, ND 55 East 100 North Suite 301 Logan, Utah   84323
Phone: 435-755-9413

Jeffrey V. Wright, ND 3311 North University Avenue Ste #100 Provo,
Utah 84604 Phone: 801-374-5677 Web: www.utahvalleyhealthclinic.com

Vermont

Sojourns Community Health Clinic 4923 U.S. Route 5 Westminster, Vermont
05158 Phone: 802-722-4023

Gabriel Tomas Archdeacon, ND 174 River St. Montpelier, Vermont   05602
Phone: 802-505-0597 Email: DrGabriel@tolmedicine.com
Web: www.ToLMedicine.com

Mary Louise Bove, ND 1063 Marlboro Rd. Brattleboro, Vermont   05301
Phone: 802-254-9332 Web: www.brattleboronaturopathic.com

Greg Burkland, ND 75 Allen Street Rutland, Vermont   05701
Phone: 802-922-6171 Email: drgreg@greenmountainND.com
Web: www.greenmountainND.com

Donna B. Caplan, ND 172 Berlin St. Montpelier, Vermont   05602
Phone: 802-229-2635 Email: donnacaplan@vtimed.com
Web: www.vtimed.com

Rebecca Chollet, ND 3804 Shelburne Rd. Shelburne, Vermont   05482
Phone: 802-985-8250 Email: dr_becky@monadnocknaturalmed.com
Web: www.vtnaturalmed.com

Samantha Kane Eagle, ND MS 205 Main Street 2nd Floor Brattleboro,
Vermont   05301 Phone: 802-275-4732
Email: info@biologichealthcare.com Web: www.biologichealthcare.com

Jus Crea Giammarino, ND 1086 Marlboro Rd Battleboro, Vermont
Phone: 802-254-9332 Web: www.brattleboronaturopathic.com

Susan B. Kowalsky, N.D. P.O. Box 851 Norwich, Vermont   05055
Phone: 802-649-1064 Web: www.DrKowalsky.com

Karen Miller-Lane, LAc ND 50 Court St. Middlebury, Vermont 05753
Phone: 802-388-6250 Web:www.naturalmedicineofvermont.com

Bernie Noe, ND 61 Elm Street Montpelier, Vermont 05602
Phone: 802-229-2038 Email: info@greenmountainhealth.com
Web: www.GreenMountainHealth.com

Lorilee Schoenbeck, ND 23 Mansfield Ave. Burlington, Vermont 05401
Phone: 802-985-8250 Web: www.DrLorilee.com

Bill Warnock, ND 3804 Shellburne Rd. Shelburne, Vermont 05482
Phone: 802-985-8250 Email: ccnm@vtnaturalmed.com
Web: www.vtnaturalmed.com

Maureen Williams, ND PO Box 185 Hartland, Vermont 05048
Phone: 802-436-3800

Virginia

White Mountain Clinic 855 N Lexington St Arlington, Virginia 22205
Phone: 202-557-1182 Web: www.whitemountainclinic.com

Valeria Birch, ND 9579 Blake Park Ct. Fairfax, Virginia 22031
Phone: 202-341-5522 Web: www.birchnaturopathic.com

Theresa L Collier, ND 5102 W. Village Green Drive Suite 103 Midlothian,
Virginia 23112 Phone: 804-744-4927 Email: bewell@cavtel.net
Web: www.theresacolliernd.com

Lynne C. David, LAc ND MSOM MS 855 N Lexington St Arlington,
Virginia 22205 Phone: 202-557-1182
Web: www.whitemountainclinic.com

Christie Fleetwood, ND RPh 11923 Centre Street Chester, Virginia 23831
Phone: 804-768-9333 Email: cffleetwood@verizon.net
Web: www.ChristieFleetwoodNDRPh.com

Christopher Johnson, ND 1423 Powhatan St Suite #7 Alexandria, Virginia
22314 Phone: 703-836-3678 Web: www.thrivenaturopathic.com

Teerawong Kasiolarn, LAc ND MS 21785 Filigree Court Ste. 100 Ashburn, Virginia 20147 Phone: 703-554-1100 x328 Email: tkasiolarn@novamedgroup.com Web: www.ndaccess.com

Deirdre Orceyre, LAc ND MSOM 140 Little Falls St Falls Church, Virginia 22046 Phone: 703-268-0862 Email: drorceyre@drorceyre.com Web: www.drorceyre.com

Deirdre Orceyre, LAc ND MSOM 140 Little Falls St Falls Church, Virginia 22046 Phone: 703-268-0862 Email: drorceyre@drorceyre.com Web: www.drorceyre.com

Floyd W. S-R Hoyt, ND PhD DHANP CNC 3305 Rivermont Ave Lynchburg, Virginia 24503 Phone: 434-851-7331 Email: Dr.Hoyt@yahoo.com

Stephanie D. Story, N.D. 1047 Angler Lane Virginia Beach, Virginia 23451
Phone: 757-428-7979 Email: sdstory2000@yahoo.com

Washington

Pure Wellness Center 10904 SE 176th St Renton, Washington 98055 Phone: 425-255-8100 x6 Web: www.purewellnesscenter.com

Bothell-Kenmore Community Health Center 6016 NE Bothell Way Suite G Kenmore, Washington 98028 Phone: 425-486-0658 Web: www.naturopathichealthservices.com

Eastside Birth Center PS 14700 NE 8th St. Bellevue, Washington 98007 Phone: 425-746-5566 Web: www.eastsidebirthcenter.com

Pure Wellness Center, ND 10904 SE 176th St. Renton, Washington 98055 Phone: 425-255-8100 x6 Web: www.PureWellnessCenters.com

Jennifer Lush, ND 2719 E Madison St suite 203 Seattle, Washington 98112 Phone: 206-568-7545 Fax: 206.568.8298 Email: drjlush@gmail.com

Kathleen Allen, ND LM 16818 140th Ave NE Woodinville, Washington 98072 Phone: 425-486-5345 Email: info@motherchildmedicine.com Web: www.motherchildmedicine.com

Kristen Allott, LAc ND , Washington   Phone: 206-579-2757
Email: allott@dynamicpaths.com Web: www.dynamicpaths.com

Rebecca Andrews, LAc ND LMT 2008 NE 65th St Seattle, Washington
98115 Phone: 206-729-0907 Email: drb@doctorbecky.net
Web: www.doctorbecky.net

Que Areste, ND MSOM 1605 12th Ave. Suite16 Seattle, Washington
98122 Phone: 206-328-2926 Email: drque@speakeasy.net

Jennifer Ash, ND 205 Clark Place SE Tumwater, Washington   98501
Phone: 360-357-1470 Email: jennifer@drjenniferash.com
Web: www.drjenniferash.com

Gary A. Bachman, ND RN 410 Commercial St #5 Mt Vernon,
Washington   98273 Phone: 360-424-3460
Email: doctorgary@nwlink.com Web: www.NaturopathicDoc.com

Karen Ball, ND 2223 112th Ave NE Suite 201 Bellevue, Washington
98004 Phone: 425-283-4928 Email: drball@seanet.com
Web: www.thesynergywellnesscenter.com

Thomas Ballard, ND RN 726 Broadway Suite 301 Seattle, Washington
98122 Phone: 206-726-0034 Email: thomasballard@speakeasy.net
Web: www.tomballardnd.com

Felice Barnow, ND 2705 E. Madison Seattle, Washington   98112
Phone: 206-328-7929 Email: info2@snabc.com

Christine Bickson, ND DHANP 2901 NE Blakeley St Seattle, Washington
98105 Phone: 206-459-1446 Email: cbickson@comcast.net

Carol Bobovski, ND 13115 121st Way NE Kirkland, Washington   98034
Phone: 425-821-1800 Email: DrB@docerenaturalhealth.com
Web: www.docerenaturalhealth.com

Cristopher Bosted, ND RN 1818 Westlake Ave. N. Ste. 304 Seattle,
Washington   98109 Phone: 206-282-2486
Email: doctorcristopher@yahoo.com

Amy Bosworth-Patton, ND 1605-116th Ave. NE Bellevue, Washington 98004 Phone: 425-451-0999 Email: dramy@redcedarwellness.com Web: www.redcedarwellness.com

Stacy Bowker, ND 1830 Bickford Ave Ste 201 Snohomish, Washington 98290 Phone: 360-282-4014 Email: drbowker@snovalleyholistic.com Web: www.snovalleyholistic.com

Heather Boyd, ND 8513 NE Hazel Dell Ave. Suite 203 Vancouver, Washington 98665 Phone: 360-573-2273 Email: nchc@nchc.info Web: www.anewme.me

Heather Boyd-Roberts, ND 8513 NE Hazel Dell Ave. Suite 203 Vancouver, Washington 98665 Phone: 360-573-2273 Email: nchc@nchc.info Web: www.anewme.me

Cindy Breed, ND 403 E Meeker #200 Kent, Washington 98030 Phone: 253-852-2866 Email: cbreed@chckc.org

Cathy Brinton, ND 7522 20th Ave NE Seattle, Washington 98115 Phone: 206-331-1396 Email: drbrinton@comcast.net Web: www.hypothyroidism-healing-options.com

Lori Brown, ND MA 2401 SE 161st Court Suite B Vancouver, Washington 98683 Phone: 360-882-1339 Web: www.naturalfamilymedicine.com

Cynthia Buxton, LAc ND 509 Olive Way Suite 1315 Seattle, Washington 98101 Phone: 206-382-9977 Email: wellness@drbuxton.com Web: www.DrBuxton.com

Cynthia Bye, ND 2400 Broadway St Vancouver, Washington 98663 Phone: 360-695-8800 Email: cbyend@yahoo.com Web: www.cynthiabye.com

Cheri Carmean, ND 8821 51st Ave NE Marysville, Washington 98270 Phone: 360-653-3140 Email: drchericarmean@msn.com Web: www.avalonwellness.net

Salina Chan, LAc ND 663 S King St Seattle, Washington 98104 Phone: 206-292-9646 Email: salina@drsalinachan.com Web: www.drsalinachan.com

Sooyoung Chun, ND 1530 140th Ave. NE #101 Bellevue, Washington 98005 Phone: 425-233-8254 Email: drsooyoung@hotmail.com Web: www.mediartfamily.com

Amy Clewell, ND 17425 Vashon Highway SW Vashon, Washington 98070
Phone: 206-408-7400 Email: dramyclewell@gmail.com

Emily Colwell, ND 3670 Stone Way North Seattle, Washington 98103 Web: www.bastyrcenter.org/content/view/1074

Sean Congdon, ND 3670 Stone Way North Seattle, Washington 98103 Phone: 206-834-4100 Web: www.bastyrcenter.org

Chris Cotner, ND 13115 121st Way NE Suite C Kirkland, Washington 98034 Phone: 425-821-1800 Email: chris@cornerstonehealthclinic.com Web: www.cornerstonehealthclinic.com

Seth Cowan, ND 916 S. 3rd St. Mount Vernon, Washington 98273 Phone: 360-336-5658 Email: info@skagitdocs.net Web: www.skagitdocs.net

Janet A Cutro, ND 2804 Grand Avenue Everett, Washington 98201 Phone: 425-258-4633 Email: drcutro@soundholitichealth.com

Nooshin K. Darvish, ND 1899 116th Ave NE Bellevue, Washington 98004
Phone: 425-451-0404 Email: info@DrDarvish.com Web: www.DrDarvish.com

Leslie DeGasparis, ND 555 116th Ave NE Bellevue, Washington 98004 Phone: 425-688-1994 Email: drleslied@comcast.net Web: www.drleslied.com

Meredith Distante, ND 532 NE Third Ave. Camas, Washington 98607 Phone: 360-834-6964 Email: dr.merrie@blossomnaturalhealth.com

Trina Doerfler, ND DC 6300 9th Ave. NE Level 2 Seattle, Washington 98115 Phone: 206-428-2075 Web: www.seattlehealingarts.com

May Eng, ND 9111 Roosevelt Way NE Seattle, Washington 98115
Phone: 206-525-8078 Web: www.naturopathichealthservices.com

Alethea Fleming, ND 1015 6th Street Suite #108 Anacortes, Washington
98221 Phone: 360-630-3022 Web: www.vitalagingclinic.com

Natalie Freedman, ND PT 3670 Stone Way N. Seattle, Washington 98103
Phone: 206-834-4100 Email: nfreedman@bastyr.edu
Web: http://bastyrcenter.org

Jill K Fresonke, ND 147 Madrone Lane N Bainbridge Island, Washington
98110 Phone: 206-780-2626 Email: JFresonke@aol.com
Web: www.biwellness.com

Marnie Frisch, ND 7935 216th St SW Edmonds, Washington 98026
Phone: 425-672-2113 Email: whnaturopathy@gmail.com
Web: www.edmondswellnessclinic.com

Carolyn M Fuller, ND Practitioner Care Seattle, Washington 98103
Phone: 206-834-4100 Email: cfuller@bastyr.edu
Web: www.bastyrcenter.org

Adam Geiger, ND 2505 S. 320th St Federal Way, Washington 98003
Phone: 253-529-3050 Email: ag@paracelsusclinic.com
Web: www.paracelsusclinic.com

Mark A Gignac, ND 122 16th Ave E 2nd Floor Seattle, Washington
98112
Phone: 206-292-2277 Email: docgignac@aol.com
Web: www.seattlecancerwellness.com

Erik William Gilbertson, ND DC Puyallup, Washington 98372
Phone: 253-845-6636 Email: gilbertson_e@yahoo.com

Jane Guiltinan, ND 3670 Stone Way North Seattle, Washington 98103
Phone: 206-834-4105 Email: jguiltin@bastyr.edu

Jana Hagen, ND 2324 Eastlake AVE E Seattle, Washington 98102
Phone: 206-734-4779 Email: dr.janahagen.nd@gmail.com
Web: www.recoveringhealth.net

Colleen Hart, N.D. 18806 Eighth Ave. S.W. Seattle, Washington 98166
Phone: 253-942-3301 Web: www.fwnmedical.com

Amy Hawkins, ND 2901 NE Blakeley Street Seattle, Washington   98105
Phone: 425-773-0420 Email: amyhawkinsnd@comcast.net

Joan Hill, ND 14419 Greenwood Ave N #321 Seattle, Washington
98133
Phone: 206-851-0875 Email: dr.joanhill.nd@comcast.net

Joanne Hillary, ND 122 N. Argonne #3 Spokane, Washington   99212
Phone: 509-924-6782 Email: hillarynd@earthlink.net

Shannon Hirst, ND 12900 NE 180th St. #100 Bothell, Washington
98011
Phone: 425-398-9355 Fax: 425-486-5913
Web: www.sammamishmedicine.com

Rebecka Hoppins Campbell, ND 19514 64th Ave W Ste B Lynnwood,
Washington   98036 Phone: 425-985-5421 Email: drhoppins@yahoo.com
Web: www.seattlenaturopathy.com

Dean Howell, ND 2840 Northup Way #104 Bellevue, Washington   98004
Phone: 888-252-0411 Email: drhowell@drdeanhowell.com
Web: www.drdeanhowell.com

Jenefer S. Huntoon, ND 1329 N 45th St. Seattle, Washington   98103
Phone: 206-632-8804 Web: www.drhuntoon.com

Angila Jaeggli, ND 1610 NE Eastgate Blvd. Ste. 250 Pullman, Washington
99163 Phone: 509-432-4301 Web: www.sagemedicineclinic.com

Laura James, ND 1601 116th Avenue NE Bellevue, Washington   98004
Phone: 425-451-0999 Email: drlaura@redcedarwellness.com
Web: www.redcedarwellness.com

Eric Jones, ND 3670 Stone Way N. Seattle, Washington   98103
Phone: 206-834-4129 Web: www.bastyr.edu

Elinor E. Jordan, ND 208 11th Avenue SE Olympia, Washington   98501
Phone: 360-491-4131 Web: www.naturalhealthclinicofolympia.com

Joseph Katzinger, ND 18021 15th Ave Ne Shoreline, Washington   98155
Phone: 206-524-1003 Email: drkatzinger@wholehealthseattle.com
Web: www.wholehealthseattle.com

Sherry J. A. Kerchner, ND 2366 Eastlake Ave. E Seattle, Washington
98102 Phone: 206-323-7864 Web: www.ahealthrenaissance.com

Keyanoosh Khorami, ND 17530 132nd Ave NE Woodinville, Washington
98072 Phone: 425-483-1200 Email: drkeya@wholisticmedical.com

Richard J. Kitaeff, LAc ND 23700 Edmonds Way Edmonds, Washington
98026 Phone: 425-775-6001 Email: newhealthmed@bigplanet.com
Web: www.newhealthmed.com

Whitney Knickrehm, ND 119 N. Commercial Street Ste.910 Bellingham,
Washington   98225 Phone: 360-738-7654 Web: www.bnfm.com

Maegan Knutson, LAc ND 17311 135th Ave NE Sute C800 Woodinville,
Washington   98072 Phone: 425-402-9999
Email: healthmoves@yahoo.com Web: www.healthmoves.org

Steven Koda, ND 9594 First Avenue NE No. 293 Seattle, Washington
98115 Email: info@VSNaturopathy.com Web: www.vsnaturopathy.com

Stella Kondilis, LAc ND 610 NW 79th Street Seattle, Washington   98117
Phone: 206-356-7526 Email: drstellak@hotmail.com
Web: www.drstella.com

Christopher J. Kozura, ND LMP 3216 N.E. 45th Place Suite 212 Seattle,
Washington   98105 Phone: 206-523-9300
Web: www.vitalitynaturally.com

Alex Kraft, LAc ND 17311 135th Ave NE Woodenville, Washington
98072
Phone: 425-402-9999 Email: dralexkraft@hotmail.com
Web: www.dralexkraft.com

Barbara Kreemer, ND DHANP 315 First Ave. W. # A Seattle, Washington
  98119 Phone: 206-281-4282 Web: www.qanc.com

Christa C. Lamothe, ND 316 Main Street Edmonds, Washington   98020
Phone: 425-361-1795 Web: www.naturopathicdermatology.com

Hillary Marisa Lampers, ND LMT 707 Pine Ave STE A102 Snohomish, Washington 98290 Phone: 360-568-7075 Email: drlampers@nwncr.com Web: www.nwncr.com

Jean Lawler, ND MA 15650 NE 24th Street Suite C-2 Bellevue, Washington 98008 Phone: 425-466-8202 Web: www.JeanLawlerND.com

Jean McFadden Layton, ND 1329 Lincoln St Suite 3 Bellingham, Washington 98229 Phone: 360-734-1659 Fax: 360-734-1659 Web: www.naturalhealthbellingham.com

Douglas C. Lewis, ND 9111 Roosevelt Way NE Seattle, Washington 98115 Phone: 206-525-8078 Email: dclewisnd@qwest.net

Brad S Lichtenstein, ND 7908 Ashworth Ave N Unit B Seattle, Washington 98103 Phone: 206-545-7133 Email: pranaplay@mac.com Web: www.pranaplay.com

Denise Linehan, ND 1140-A 140th Ave NE Bellevue, Washington 98005 Phone: 425-957-0761 Web: www.mybcfh.com

Molly A. Linton, ND 1409 NW 85th St. Seattle, Washington 98117 Phone: 206-781-2206 Email: d2rmolly@aol.com Web: www.emeraldcityclinic.com

Brandy Lipscomb, ND P.O. Box 1568 Sultan, Washington 98294 Phone: 360-793-0206 Email: info@skyrivernaturalhealth.com Web: www.skyrivernaturalhealth.com

Angela London, ND 2376 Main Street Suite 3 Ferndale, Washington 98248 Phone: 360-384-2900 Email: Londonhealthcenter@verizon.net Web: www.londonhealthcenterinc.com

Heidi Lucas, ND 122 16th Ave East Seattle, Washington 98112 Phone: 206-292-2277 Web: www.seattlecancerwellness.com

Dan Lukaczer, ND Fife, Washington 98424 Phone: 253-926-2222 Email: doc@danlukaczernd.com

Janile Martin, LAc ND RN 1605 116th Ave. NE #108 Bellevue, Washington 98004 Phone: 425-451-0999
Email: drjanilemartin@hotmail.com

Tennille Marx, ND 9827 NE 120th Pl. Kirkland, Washington 98034
Phone: 425-820-2800 Email: drmarx1@hotmail.com
Web: www.healthybody-healthymind.com

Tammy McInnis, ND 2830 228th Avenue SE Suite C Sammamish, Washington 98075 Phone: 425-557-8900
Email: tmcinnis@naturomedica.com Web: www.naturomedica.com

Leah J. McNeill, ND 2025 112th Ave NE Bellevue, Washington 98004
Phone: 425-452-9366 Email: leahmcneill@msn.com
Web: www.NaturalMedicineForHealth.com

Steven Milkis, ND 3670 Stone Way N. Seattle, Washington 98103
Phone: 206-834-4148 Email: smilkis@bastyr.edu

Eva Miller, ND 6300 9th Ave NE Seattle, Washington 98115
Phone: 206-522-5646 Email: emiller@seattlehealingarts.com

Melissa H Minoff, LAc ND 6300 9th Ave NE Suite 310 Seattle, Washington 98115 Phone: 206-524-0863 Email: mhminoff@gmail.com

Leah Mitchell, ND LM 853 NE 68th Street Seattle, Washington 98115
Phone: 206-284-6040 Web: www.mitchell-center.com

Jill Monster, ND 2830 228th Ave. SE Sammamish, Washington 98075
Phone: 425-557-8900 Email: jmonster@naturomedica.com
Web: www.naturomedica.com

Willow Moore, ND DC 11930 SW Greenburg Rd Tigard, Washington 97223 Phone: 502-639-1712 Email: drwillowmoore@yahoo.com
Web: www.tigardholistic.com

Willow Moore, ND DC 11930 SW Greenburg Rd Tigard, Washington 97223 Phone: 502-639-1712 Email: drwillowmoore@yahoo.com
Web: www.tigardholistic.com

Cornelia Moynihan, LAc ND 201 N. 'T' Street Tacoma, Washington 98403
Phone: 253-250-2630 Email: drcornelia@gmail.com

Elissa Mullen, ND 5617 California Ave SW Seattle, Washington
Phone: 206-388-2929 Email: drelissa@seattlewellnessprograms.com
Web: www.seattlewllnessprograms.com

Michael T. Murray, ND 18304 NW Montreux Drive Issaquah, Washington
98207 Email: doctormurray@doctormurray.com

Tara B. Brooke Nelson, ND 4744 41st Avenue SW #102 Seattle,
Washington 98114 Phone: 206-932-0880 Email: tnelson@bastyr.edu
Web: www.doctortarabrooke.com

Erica Oberg, ND 1600 E Jefferson St. Ste 603 Seattle, Washington 98122
Phone: 206-726-0034 Web: www.icmedicine.com

Catherine Orsi, ND LMT 4746 44th Ave SW Seattle, Washington 98116
Phone: 206-938-9355 Email: docorsi@quidnunc.net

Emily Penney, ND 1233 Lawrence St Port Townsend, Washington 98368
Phone: 360-385-2107 Email: info@tolwc.com Web: www.tolwc.com

Jena Peterson, ND 2008 NE 65th Street Seattle, Washington 98115
Phone: 206-729-0907 Email: drjenand@yahoo.com

Gary Piscopo, LAc ND 430 Elva Way East Wenatchee, Washington
98802
Phone: 509-886-9355 Web: www.alpinebewell.com

Joseph E. Pizzorno, ND 4220 NE 135th Street Seattle, Washington 98125
Phone: 206-361-4620 Email: drpizzorno@salugenecists.com
Web: www.drpizzorno.com

Richard Posmantur, LAc ND 2705 E. Madison Seattle, Washington 98112
Phone: 206-328-7929 Email: info@snabc.com Web: www.snabc.com

Caryn Potenza, ND LMT 1137 W. Garland Ave Spokane, Washington
99205 Phone: 509-327-5143 Email: drpotenza@windroseclinic.com
Web: www.windroseclinic.com

David G. Ramaley, ND DC DACNB 11050- 5th Ave. NE # 205 Seattle,
Washington 98121 Phone: 206-306-7797
Web: www.seattlenaturalhealth.com

Karen Pantilat Rasmussen, ND LM 900 S. 336th Street Federal Way, Washington 98003 Phone: 253-942-3301 Web: www.fwnmedical.com

Judyth L. Reichenberg-Ullman, ND MSW 131 3rd Ave. N Edmonds, Washington 98020 Phone: 425-774-5599
Web: www.healthyhomeopathy.com

Adam Rinde, ND 11520 NE 20th St. Bellevue, Washington 98004
Phone: 425-736-1252 Fax: 425-269-6947
Email: info@soundintegrative.com Web: www.soundintegrative.com

Heidi J Robel, LAc ND 307 S. 12th Ave STE 11 Yakima, Washington 98902
Phone: 509-469-2483 Email: drheidirobel@hotmail.com
Web: www.drheidirobel.com

Scott D. Rose, LAc ND 607 Market Street Kirkland, Washington 98033
Phone: 425-822-8356 Email: DrRose@AndersonNaturalHealth.com
Web: www.AndersonNaturalHealth.com

Robin Russell, ND 12911 - 120th Ave NE Kirkland, Washington 98034
Phone: 425-820-7700 Email: dr.robin@naturalpediatricmedicine.com
Web: www.naturalpediatricmedicine.com

Wendy Alisa Schloss, ND 4852 37th Ave South Seattle, Washington 98118 Phone: 206-725-3636 Email: drwendy@holistichealthpartners.org
Web: www.holistichealthpartners.org

Aurora Sedmak, ND 4259 E Lk Samm Shore Ln SE Sammamish, Washington 98075 Phone: 206-910-8236
Email: drsedmak@transformational-health.com
Web: www.transformational-health.com

Trina Seligman, ND 11520 NE 20th St. Bellevue, Washington 98004
Phone: 425-646-4747 Web: www.eimed.com

Emily Sharpe, ND 1707 F Street Bellingham, Washington 98225
Phone: 360-734-1560 Email: naturalhealthclinic@yahoo.com
Web: www.members.aol.com/fstreetnhc/

Kevin D Shaw, LAc ND MSOM 2804 Grand Avenue Everett, Washington 98201 Phone: 425-258-4633 Email: info@soundholistichealth.com
Web: www.soundholistichealth.com

Laura A. Shelton, ND 1707 F Street Bellingham, Washington   98225
Phone: 360-734-1560 Web: www.fstreetnaturalhealthclinic.com

Lorina Shinsato, ND 11415 NE 128th St. Ste. 130 Kirkland, Washington
98034 Phone: 425-273-0741
Email: Dr.Shinsato@primavitamedicine.com

Michelle Simon, ND PhD 6300 9th Avenue NE Ste. 310 Seattle,
Washington 98115 Phone: 206-524-0863
Email: msimon@seattlehealingarts.com Web: www.drmichellesimon.com

Suzanne L. Sykurski, ND MS LMP 1180 NW Maple St. Suite 140
Issaquah, Washington 98027 Phone: 425-391-1433
Email: alpinenaturopathic@yahoo.com Web: www.avikai.com

Jacqueline Thomas, ND 430 Elva Way East Wenatchee, Washington
98802 Phone: 509-886-9355 Web: www.alpinebewell.com

Sarah Tung, LAc ND 222 Kenyon St. NW Olympia, Washington   98502
Phone: 360-350-9014 Email: drsarahtung@gmail.com
Web: www.PacificNaturalHealthcare.com

Ruth Urand, ND 20270 Front Street NE #202 Poulsbo, Washington
98370 Phone: 360-598-6999 Email: drurand@embarqmail.com
Web: www.drurand.com

Jamey Wallace, ND 3670 Stone Way North Seattle, Washington   98103
Phone: 206-834-4141 Web: www.bastyrcenter.org

Laura C Walton, ND LMT 1409 NW 85th St. Seattle, Washington
98117
Phone: 206-781-2206 Email: laura@vitalityhealthcare.net
Web: www.emeraldcityclinic.com

Stephen Wangen, ND 1229 Madison St. Ste.1220 Seattle, Washington
98104 Phone: 206-264-1111 or 888-546-6
Email: info@ibstreatmentcenter.com
Web: www.IBSTreatmentcenter.com

Letitia M. Watrous, ND 1137 W. Garland Ave. Spokane, Washington 99205 Phone: 509-327-5143 Email: LWatrousND@aol.com Web: www.windroseclinic.com

Brandy Webb, ND 6720 Eastside Dr. NE Tacoma, Washington 98422 Phone: 253-952-2776 Web: www.sagenatural.com

Joseph Wessels 1903 D St. Bellingham, Washington 98225 Phone: 360-734-9500 Email: jwessels@earthlink.net

Karyn N White, ND 145 Lilly Rd NE Suite 102 Olympia, Washington 98506 Phone: 360-357-7902 Email: Drkarynwhite@yahoo.com

Melanie Whittaker, ND RN 9902-270th St. NW Ste. A Stanwood, Washington 98292 Phone: 360-629-2222 Web: www.altmedclinic.com

Katherine Wiggin, ND 2400 Broadway St. Ste. #7 Vancouver, Washington 98663 Phone: 503-449-1167 Email: drkate@drkatewiggin.com Web: www.drkatewiggin.com

Katherine Wiggin, ND 2400 Broadway St. Ste. #7 Vancouver, Washington 98663 Phone: 503-449-1167 Email: drkate@drkatewiggin.com Web: www.drkatewiggin.com

Cheryl L. Wood, ND 19031 33rd Ave. W. Ste. 301 Lynnwood, Washington 98036 Phone: 425-778-5673 Email: info@trinityclinic.com Web: www.trinityclinic.com

David B Wood, ND 19031 33rd Ave. W. Ste. 301 Lynnwood, Washington 98036 Phone: 4215-778-5673 Email: info@trinityclinic.com Web: www.trinityclinic.com

Kelly C Wright, ND 18913 Vashon Hwy SW Vashon, Washington 98070 Phone: 206-463-4778 Web: www.vashonnaturalmedicine.com

Rebecca Wynsome, ND 150 Nickerson Street Seattle, Washington 98109 Phone: 206-283-1383 Email: Clinicmgr@naturopathic.com Web: www.Naturopathic.com

Eric L. Yarnell, ND 3216 NE 45th Place Seattle, Washington 98105 Phone: 206-526-7026 Email: health@dryarnell.com Web: www.dryarnell.com

Rhian Young, ND 328 West Main Street Monroe, Washington 98272
Phone: 360-794-4500 Email: dr.rhianyoung_nd@yahoo.com
Web: www.purityintegrativehealth.com

Thomas J. Young, ND DC 8909 Gravelly Lake Dr. SW Tacoma,
Washington 98499 Phone: 253-584-1144 Web: www.youngdcnd.com

Christine Zach, ND 1736 NE Riddell Rd. Ste 103 Bremerton, Washington
98310 Phone: 360-475-0400
Email: doctorzach@kitsapnaturalmedicine.com

Jared L. Zeff, LAc ND 508 NE 139th Street Vancouver, Washington
98685
Phone: 360-823-8121 Email: DrZeff@AOL.com

Wisconsin

Allison Becker, LAc ND MSOM 4539 Woodgate Drive Suite A Janesville,
Wisconsin 53546 Phone: 608-531-0079
Web: www.naturopathicfamilyclinic.com

Bradley Bush, ND 373 280th Street Osceola, Wisconsin 54020
Phone: 603-623-6800 Email: bradley@bushnd.com
Web: www.nhnatural.com

Mihal Davis, LAc ND 602 Water Street Prairie du Sac, Wisconsin 53578
Phone: 608-588-4464 Email: mihaldavis@hotmail.com

Robin A. DiPasquale, ND 34 Apple Hill Circle Madison, Wisconsin
53717
Phone: 608-203-5890 Email: robindipasquale@yahoo.com

Jill Evenson, ND 4539 Woodgate Drive Janesville, Wisconsin 53546
Phone: 608-531-0079 Email: info@naturopathicfamilyclinic.com
Web: www.naturopathicfamilyclinic.com

Aaron Henkel, ND 4539 Woodgate Dr. Janesville, Wisconsin 53546
Phone: 608-531-0079 Email: info@naturopathicfamilyclinic.com
Web: www.naturopathicfamilyclinic.com

Michele A. Nickels, ND W62 N225 Washington Ave Cedarburg, Wisconsin 53012 Phone: 262-376-1150 Web: www.drnickels.com

Kim E. Saxe, ND 11803 W. North Ave. Wauwatosa, Wisconsin 53226 Phone: 414-258-5522 Web: www.milwaukeenaturopathic.com

Crystal Urban, LAc ND MSOM 109 S. Main Street Eagle River, Wisconsin 54521 Phone: 715-477-2431
Email: dr.crystalurban@verizon.net

ENDNOTES & REFERENCES

[1] Raghavan, A. Srinivasan, V. & Snow, K. Hypoglycemia. M*edscape.com*. Retrieved May 15 2009 from http://emedicine.medscape.com/article/122122-overview

[2] Brun JF, et. al Ibid.

[3] Harris S. Hyperinsulinism and dysinsulinism. *J Amer Med Ass,* 1924, *83,* 729-733.

[4] Lefèbvre PJ. Heurs et malheurs de l'hyperglycémie provoquée par voie orale. In: Journées Annuelles de Diabétologie de l'Hôtel-Dieu, 1987. Flammarion Médecine-Sciences, *Paris,* 313-322

and

Lefèbvre PJ, Andreani D., Marks V, Creutzfeld W. Statement on postprandial a or reactive a hypoglycaemia (Letter). *Diabetes Care,* 1988, *11,* 439.

[5] Baumel, S. *Dealing with depression naturally.* Lincolnwood, Illinois: Keats Publishing. 2000

[6] Brun JF, Fedou C, Mercier J. Postprandial Reactive Hypoglycemia. *Diabetes Metab.* 2000 Nov;26(5):337-51.

[7] Hofeldt FD. Reactive hypoglycemia. *Metabolism,* 1975, *24,* 1193-1208.

[8] Charles MA, Hofeldt F, Shackelford A. Comparison of oral glucose tolerance tests and mixed meals in patients with apparent

idiopathic post-absorptive hypoglycemia. *Diabetes,* 1981, *30,* 465-470.

[9] Brun JF, Fedou C, Mercier J. Postprandial Reactive Hypoglycemia. *Diabetes Metab.* 2000 Nov;26(5):337-51.

[10] Johnson DD, Door KE, Swenson WM, Service FJ. Reactive hypoglycemia.*JAMA,* 1980, *243,* 1151-1155.

[11] Pfeiffer, C. *Mental and Elemental Nutrients: a physician's guide to nutrition and health care.* New Canaan, CT: Keats Publishing, 1975.

[12] Raine, A. (1993). *The psychopathology of crime: Criminal behavior as a clinical disorder.* San Diego, CA: Academic Press.

[13] Brun JF, Fédou C, Bouix O, Raynaud E, Orsetti A. Evaluation of a standardized hyperglucidic breakfast test in postprandial reactive hypoglycaemia. *Diabetologia,* 1995, *38,* 494-501.

[14] Brun JF, Fédou C, Bouix O, Raynaud E, Orsetti A. Evaluation of a standardized hyperglucidic breakfast test in postprandial reactive hypoglycaemia. *Diabetologia,* 1995, *38,* 494-501.

[15] Lev-Ran A, Anderson RW. The diagnosis of postprandial Hypoglycemia. Diabetes, 1981, 30, 996-999

[16] Just one example (there are many): Buss RW, Kawsal PC, Roddam RF. Mixed meal tolerance test and reactive hypoglycemia. *Horm Metab Res,* 1982, *14,* 281-283.

[17] Brun JF, Ibid. See also Johnson DD, Door KE, Swenson WM, Service FJ. Reactive hypoglycemia. *JAMA*, 1980, *243*, 1151-1155.

[18] Below 50mg/dL may indicate a more serious problem.

[19] Harris,P. et. al. *Endocrinology in clinical practice*. London: Martin Dunitz Ltd. 2003. p.475 and Lippincott Williams and Wilkins, *Professional Guide to Diseases*. 2009.

[20] Cryer PE, Binder C, Bolli GB, Cherrington AD, Gale EAM, Gerich JE, Sherwin RS. Hypoglycemia in IDDM. *Diabetes*, 1989, *38*, 1193-1199.

[21] Brun JF, et.al. Ibid.

[22] Photo by Dawn Ashley@Flickr

[23] Açbay O,et. al.. Helicobacter pylori-induced gastritis may contribute to occurrence of postprandial symptomatic hypoglycemia.. Dig Dis Sci. 1999 Sep;44(9):1837-42.

[24] Luyckx AS, Lefèbvre PJ. Plasma insulin in reactive hypoglycemia. *Diabetes*, 1971, *20*, 435-442.

[25] Owada K, et.al. Highly increased insulin secretion in a patient with postprandial hypoglycemia: role of glucagon-like peptide-1 (7-36) amide. *Endocr J*, 1995, *42*, 147-151.

[26] Brun,JF ibid.

[27] Letiexhe MR, Scheen AJ, Gérard PL, Desaive C, Lefèbvre PJ. Insulin secretion, clearance and action before and after gastroplasty in severely obese subjects. *Int J Obes Relat Metab Disord,* 1994, *18,* 295-300 and Goodpaster BH, Kelley DE, Wing RR, Meier A, Thaete FL. Effects of weight loss on regional fat distribution and insulin sensitivity in obesity. *Diabetes,* 1999, *48,* 839-847.

[28] Raynaud E, Perez Martin A, Brun JF, Fedou C, Mercier J. Insulin sensitivity measured with the minimal model is higher in moderately overweight women with predominantly lower body fat. *Horm Metab Res,* 1999, *31,* 415-417.

[29] Chen M, Bergman RN, Porte D Jr. Insulin resistance and b-cell dysfunction in aging: the importance of dietary carbohydrate. *J Clin Endocrinol Metab,* 1988, *67,* 951-957.

[30] As cited in Baumel, S. *Dealing with depression naturally.* Lincolnwood Illinois: Keats Publishing. 2000

[31] O'Keefe SJD, Marks V. Lunchtime gin and tonic: a cause of reactive hypoglycaemia. *Lancet,* 1977, *i,* 1286-1288.

[32] Fabrykant M, Pacella BL. The association of spontaneous hypoglycemia with hypocalcemia and electro-cerebral dysfunction. *Proc Am Diab Assoc,* 1947, *7,* 233-236

[33] Heinrich Heine University of Dusseldorf. Article posted on website *University of Dusseldorf. Retirved May 18* 2009 from http://www.uni-

duesseldorf.de/MedFak/insulinoma/english%20homepage/main
page/subpage/Epostpran_hypo.htm#top

[34] Service JF. Hypoglycemic disorders. *N Engl J Med,* 1995, *332,*1144-
1152.

[35] Chalew SA, Mc Laughlin JV, Mersey JH, Adams AJ, Cornblath M,
Kowarski A. The use of the plasma epinephrine response in the
diagnosis of idiopathic postprandial syndrome. *JAMA,* 1984,
*251,*612-615.

[36] Zonera Ashraf Ali, MD, and Klaus Radebold, MD, PhD. Retrieved
May 15 2009 from:
http://emedicine.medscape.com/article/283039-overview

[37] Donaldson, David. *Psychiatric Disorders With a Chemical Basic.* Informa
Health Care, 1998

[38] Brun JF et. al. Ibid.

[39] Stein,J. *Internal Medicine.* St. Louis, Missouri: Mosby, Inc, 1998.

[40] Brun, JF et. al, Ibid.

[41] Lefebvre PJ. Hypoglycemia or non-hypoglycemia. In: Rifkin H, Colwell
JA, Taylor SI (eds) Diabetes 1991. Proceedings of the 14th
International Diabetes Federation Congress, Washington DC,
June 1991. Excerpta Medica *Amsterdam London New York Tokyo,*
1991, 757-761.

[42] Christensen, L. et. al. Dietary alteration of somatic symptoms and regional brain electrical activity. *Biological Psychiatry*. 29 (7). 1991. Pp. 679-682

[43] , S. *Dealing with depression naturally*. Lincolnwood, Illinois: Keats Publishing. 2000

[44] Airola, P. *Hypoglycemia: A better approach*. Phoenix, Arizona: Health Plus Publishers, 1977.

[45] Lefèbvre PJ. Hypoglycemia: post-prandial or reactive. *Current therapy in Endocrinology and Metabolism,* 1988, *3,* 339-341, and Lefèbvre PJ. Hypoglycemia or non-hypoglycemia. *Acta Clinica Belgica,*

[46] As advocated by JF Brun, ibid.

[47] Malaisse, W. et. al. Effects of Artificial Sweeteners on Insulin Release and Cationic Fluxes in Rat Pancreatic Islets. Laboratory of Experimental Medicine, Brussels Free University, 808 Route de Lennik, B-1070 Brussels, Belgium

[48] Brun, JF ibid

[49] Yamamoto T, Oya Y, Furusawa Y, Nonaka I, Murata M. Successful treatment of recurrent hypoglycemia by pioglitazone in a patient with myotonic dystrophy] [Article in Japanese]Rinsho Shinkeigaku. 2009 Oct;49(10):641-5.[

[50] Mirouze J, Pham TC, Selam JL, Bringer J, Chenon D. Posthyperglycaemic hypoglycaemia: effects of somatostatin. *Nouv Presse Med,* 1981, *10,* 2947-2949.

[51] Duyff, R.*American Dietetic Association complete food and nutrition guide.* Hoboken, NJ: Wiley & Sons. 2006.

INDEX

Made in the USA
Monee, IL
03 November 2019